A Guide to
Diabetes

A Guide to
Diabetes

Katherine Wright

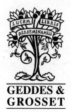

**GEDDES &
GROSSET**

Published 2003 by Geddes & Grosset,
David Dale House, New Lanark, ML11 9DJ

© 2003 Geddes & Grosset

Text by Katherine Wright

ISBN 1 84205 155 5

Printed and bound in the UK

CONTENTS

Contents

Contents

1

WHAT IS DIABETES?

Diabetes is a condition about which most people have a certain amount of knowledge or, at least, a set of beliefs that may or may not be true. For many, this extends no further than knowing that diabetes is caused by having too much sugar in the blood, the remedy for which is to take, on a regular basis, tablets or a substance called insulin which has to be injected. While this is broadly correct as far as it goes, other common beliefs, such as that diabetes is caused by eating too many sweets, are entirely mistaken! Most people know someone – a relative, friend, work colleague or acquaintance – who has diabetes. We may be aware that the person has to eat regularly but mostly avoids sweet foods and that he (or she) carries medication about with him. Perhaps we also know that the person sometimes has to check his sugar levels by carrying out blood glucose tests at home.

Of course, if you yourself, or a close member of your family, is already affected by diabetes, you will know a great deal more than this. However, it is vital that we should all be better informed, whether we are at present directly affected or not, for one very important reason. This is the fact that the incidence of both of the two main categories of diabetes is increasing. In particular, the number of people affected by the main form of the condition is soaring, not only in the UK but in many other countries as well. It is set to reach epidemic proportions and to rank alongside illnesses such as AIDS in presenting a huge challenge to public health on a global scale. If you or someone close to you develops diabetes, the more you understand about the condition, the better prepared you can be. The aim of this book is to try and help increase that understanding, by presenting an overview of the many aspects of this complex disorder. Of course, the first source of information and guidance for people with diabetes is the clinical diabetes team involved in their care. But it is further hoped that the information included here will support that given by medical experts and provide a useful source of reference for individuals and their families affected by diabetes.

In the following pages, for convenience, topics are introduced and discussed under a series of headings. However, even medical experts and scientists have found that diabetes is not a condition that fits neatly into categories. It can be likened to the overlapping and intersecting circles of ripples that occur when pebbles are thrown into a pool of water. Inevitably one aspect overlaps with and affects another, and in addition the treatment, control and management of an individual's diabetes change with time and circumstance. Hence, where necessary, a topic may appear under more than one heading. Finally, although there are facts, symptoms and known potential consequences associated with this condition, perhaps the most important aspect is that each person's diabetes is unique. In the majority of cases of newly diagnosed diabetes, even the most experienced specialist would not wish to predict the future health of the person concerned. Many individual factors – physical, psychological and emotional – affect the way in which people manage and cope with their diabetes. The good news is that most are able to lead long, active and fulfilling lives, just like anyone else and the whole emphasis in modern treatment is to enable those with diabetes to do just that. The Olympic athlete Sir Steve Redgrave, winner of five gold medals for rowing, is on record as saying that he believed his career was over when he was diagnosed with diabetes. However, with the encouragement of his consultant and diabetes care team, he went on to fulfil his greatest ambition in the Sydney Olympics in the year 2000.

The Background to Diabetes: Insulin, Glucose and the Provision of Energy

Diabetes mellitus is most correctly defined as a series of disorders or a syndrome in which the body is unable to properly regulate the processing, or metabolism, of carbo-hydrates, fats and proteins. It is caused by an absolute or partial deficiency of the important hormone insulin, which is produced and released by specialized cells (known as beta cells) located in the pancreas. The pancreas itself is a gland that is situated between the duodenum and the spleen and behind the stomach and is about 15 cm in length. It contains two main types of cells both of which produce secretions. The first group secretes digestive enzymes involved in the breakdown of food, and the second comprises clusters of cells called the islets of Langerhans, which produce hormones. As noted above, the beta cells are the ones that produce and release insulin but others, the alpha cells, secrete a different hormone called gluca-gon which is also involved in the regulation of blood glu-cose levels. Glucagon acts principally upon processes that occur in the liver (*see* below) and has an important role in preventing hypoglycaemia. Hypoglycaemia is one of the main features of the form of diabetes that require insulin treatment and is described in greater detail in Chapter 6.

The function of insulin is to regulate the levels of glucose (the body's energy source) in the blood in order to ensure that enough is made available at all times to all the various tissues and organs, so that vital life-processes can continue. Glucose is the simplest form of sugar molecule, being the end product of carbohydrate digestion and the form in which carbohydrate is absorbed from the gut into the bloodstream. Hence the main and ultimate source of glucose is carbohydrate taken in as food, but the body does not rely on this alone. When dietary glucose is in short supply, the body turns to alternative sources and processes. An understanding of the regulatory mechanisms involving insulin is important in order to comprehend what happens in diabetes, and so it is useful to look briefly at these in a little more detail.

Insulin has short-term (metabolic) and longer-term activity within the body, both of which affect other processes important to health. Returning to the analogy of ripples in a pool, when something goes wrong with the activity of insulin, as in diabetes, the effects can be far-reaching and at first sight, perhaps somewhat surprising. It is these 'ripple effects' that are responsible for some of the potential, LONG-TERM COMPLICATIONS OF DIABETES that are discussed in Chapters 8 and 9.

Insulin is released from the beta cells in response to certain triggers, in particular, the presence of glucose in the blood which rises following digestion of meals containing carbohydrate. Other triggers are the presence of *amino acids* (the end products of protein digestion) and certain hormones, including glucagon, released from the pancreatic alpha cells. Release of insulin is inhibited by the presence of certain other hormones, especially *adrenaline* and *noradrenaline*, produced by the *adrenal glands*, which are also known as catecholamines, and also somatostatin. Adrenaline is the hormone that prepares the body for 'fright, flight or fight' and is sometimes called the stress hormone, while somatostatin is produced by a third type of islet of Langerhans cells, the delta cells. In addition, it is possible that a high release of insulin may itself inhibit further secretion of the hormone.

Once released, insulin carries out its effects by acting within cells. The insulin molecules do this by each attaching to a specialized receptor site located in the cell *membrane* that is tailor-made to receive it. All human cells contain a number of insulin receptors but some have a particular affinity for the hormone. These are: adipocytes (fat cells); hepatocytes (liver cells); skeletal myocytes (voluntary muscle cells, i.e. those attached to bones and joints). The affinity of these target cells for insulin becomes more meaningful when the overall regulatory activity of the hormone is understood, and this is described below. The effects of insulin take place by means of a whole series of biochemical events that begin to be activated once the insulin molecules are locked into place on their receptors. These are known as post-binding or post-receptor events (because they occur after the insulin molecules are bound to their receptors). They take place within cells, that is, on the inner side of the cell membrane. They are highly complex biochemical reactions involving enzymes, transport mechanisms and even, ultimately, the expression or working of certain *genes* (one of the longer-term effects of insulin). While it is not necessary to know how these reactions work, a knowledge of their existence and that of insulin receptors is quite important in understanding diabetes.

Insulin is the principal regulator of blood glucose and this is achieved through its actions being subjected to certain checks and balances, producing a system which in normal health is very finely tuned and controlled. The checks and balances operate mainly at post-receptor level, that is, within cells and they mainly involve counter-regulatory hormones which act antagonistically (i.e. against) the effects of insulin. The most important of these is glucagon, and also significant is *growth hormone*, secreted by the *thyroid gland*.

In normal health, insulin is produced at a low level throughout any 24-hour period, accounting for about half of the total amount released. However, as mentioned above, this increases markedly when blood glucose levels rise following digestion of a carbohydrate-containing meal, and insulin then goes to work to remove this from the circulation. It does this by promoting the uptake of glucose by all cells to fulfil their immediate energy needs. Also, and most important, it promotes the removal of glucose to liver and skeletal muscle cells, where it is converted to *glycogen*. Glycogen or animal starch is a complex carbohydrate molecule and is the body's main reserve energy store, which can be drawn upon in times of need. Additionally, insulin stimulates the uptake of surplus glucose by fatty tissue where it is converted to *triglyceride* (a type of fat) molecules and stored. Insulin has other effects as well but in order to understand these, it is necessary to look at what happens in the liver. We also need to examine the chain of events that occurs when carbohydrate and food in general are in short supply. If food is unavailable, there is no need for high levels of insulin to be released, but the body still requires glucose to supply its energy needs. In these circumstances, for example after the nightly fast, a process called glycogenolysis takes place in the liver in which glycogen is broken down into glucose and released into the circulation. The hormone which stimulates this process is glucagon. In addition, and especially when glycogen stores have themselves been depleted and there is still a lack of food, another mechanism called gluconeogenesis is activated. In this process, stored fats and eventually proteins are broken down and the molecules released are used by the liver to manufacture glucose. Breakdown (or *lipolysis*) of triglycerides also takes place in fatty tissues and releases fatty acids. In the liver these are utilized to make glucose, but another process called *ketogenesis* (which has potentially serious consequences in diabetes) also occurs as a result of this process. Ketogenesis produces molecules called *ketone bodies* or *ketones* which, in normal conditions as described above, provide energy for outlying tissues such as muscles. A familiar ketone body and one which is important in diabetes, is acetone, which has a characteristic 'fruity', 'peardrops' aroma. One of the most important functions of insulin, and one which is critical in diabetes, is to suppress both the breakdown of triglycerides and ketogenesis. The body's normal energy stores – glycogen and then triglycerides – are used first when food is unavailable. But if fasting continues, proteins derived from tissues such as the muscles eventually have to be utilized and converted, by gluconeogenesis, into glucose. Glycogenolysis and gluconeogenesis occur when insulin levels are low because the body has not received an intake of food. In normal circumstances, the body has enough reserves of stored energy to 'fuel' its daily activity, and protein does not need to be utilized for this purpose. Any protein eaten can therefore be used for its

17

normal purposes of tissue growth and repair. Insulin indirectly regulates the fate of protein through its effects upon carbohydrates and fats. The processes described above determine what happens when a person embarks upon a weight-loss diet or a 'fad' diet such as a protein-only regime and, as we shall see, are highly significant in diabetes. In normal health, insulin and its counter-regulatory system are so finely tuned that they maintain blood glucose levels within an extremely narrow range of 3–8 mmol/l (millimols per litre).

Defining and Diagnosing Diabetes

The information given above is designed to provide a better understanding of diabetes and the reasons behind its symptoms and manifestations. As noted previously, diabetes is caused by a complete or partial deficiency of insulin or a lack of its effects. Hence the defect may be in the production and release of the hormone or it may occur at receptor or post-receptor level. The second situation is known as INSULIN RESISTANCE and the problem may lie with the receptors themselves or with post-receptor events. If the receptors themselves are involved, it may be because they are too few in number or because they have lost some of their ability to bind to insulin. Defects in insulin receptors can sometimes be corrected with treatment, but in very rare cases they may be a part of a severe, inherited condition. Malfunction in post-receptor events preventing insulin from performing its normal metabolic actions is quite common. Usually, there is a degree of impairment, so that the actions of insulin are rendered less effective, rather than a complete breakdown of the system. Post-receptor defects are highly complex, may not be reversible, and are a prominent feature in the most common form of diabetes, TYPE 2 DIABETES. The other main reason for insulin deficiency has to do with defects in the pancreatic beta cells of the islets of Langerhans.

Whatever the reason, or combination of reasons, behind the deficiency of insulin, the effect is to cause a sustained rise in the level of blood glucose or *hyperglycaemia*. An elevated level of blood sugar is the defining feature of diabetes mellitus but this does not always produce a clear-cut set of symptoms. The syndrome ranges from producing no symptoms at all to severe illness due to acute and potentially fatal metabolic complications. In general, severity of symptoms is related to the degree of insulin deficiency, although there are other factors which may influence this. One of the functions of insulin is regulation of the normal salts/water balance. Hyperglycaemia may result in glucose entering the urine and disruption of the body's normal electrolytes (salts) to water ratios in the tissues. A feature of this imbalance is that the person passes an abnormally large quantity of urine (*polyuria*), and this may be particularly the case during the night (nocturia). Excessive urination leads to further loss of salts such as sodium and potassium and an increased thirst, so that the person drinks excessively. Increased urination, thirst and excessive drinking in diabetes may be medically referred to as osmotic symptoms. The presence of sugar in the urine quite commonly encourages opportunistic infections by yeast organisms (thrush), with irritation and itching around the external opening of the *urethra*. High glucose levels in the blood can affect the lens of the eye which may become swollen, causing inability to focus and a blurring of vision. This is a temporary and reversible situation which is rectified with treatment for the diabetes, as distinct from DIABETIC RETINOPATHY which is a potential LONG-TERM COMPLICATION of the syndrome. Other symptoms that are quite common in diabetes include recurrent infections such as boils, mood swings and irritability, and a tingling 'pins and needles' sensation in the feet and hands.

If deficiency in insulin continues to be severe, the mechanisms described in the previous section accelerate as fat and protein are broken down in the liver's attempt to provide the body with energy. As a result, blood glucose levels rise even higher, but the continuing lack of insulin means that the body remains deprived of energy. Symptoms of this include extreme tiredness and rapid weight loss. In serious cases, as a result of ketogenesis, *ketosis* or acidosis occurs and there is a build up of ketones in the blood, from which they pass into the urine (*ketonuria*). There may be a detectable smell of acetone from the person's breath. In extreme and severe untreated cases, there may be a progression to a serious and potentially fatal condition called DIABETIC KETOACIDOSIS (DKA), which is described in Chapter 7.

Many people are newly diagnosed with diabetes each day in the UK. Although some will have gone to their doctor feeling unwell or with symptoms that have indicated diabetes, for many others the diagnosis comes as a complete surprise. This is because it is quite common for diabetes to be detected during a routine health check or during a period of hospitalization for some other problem. Quite often, initial suspicion of diabetes is raised when sugar is found to be present in a urine sample. However, further testing of blood samples is needed for the diagnosis to be confirmed. It is estimated that 50 per cent of those with the commonest form of diabetes – as many as one million people – are at present undiagnosed and unaware that they have the syndrome. It is probable that many of these people either have no symptoms or that symptoms have developed so slowly and insidiously that they have not recognized that anything is amiss. Ultimately, diagnosis is usually made by testing one or more samples of venous blood (from veins) or *plasma*. Samples may need to be given on more than one day, depending, to some extent, on whether the person is exhibiting any other symptoms of diabetes. In Britain the diagnostic criteria established by the World Health Organization (WHO) in 1980 and 1985 are still in use, although these have since been challenged and revised by the American Diabetes Association (ADA) through their Expert Committee on the Diagnosis and Classification of Diabetes Mellitus, 1997. These criteria are as follows.

- WHO: A level of glucose at or exceeding 11.1 mmol/l in the plasma of venous blood sampled at random. (Or 10.1 mmol/l if whole venous blood is sampled.)

  OR

  A fasting glucose level at or exceeding 7.8 mmol/l in the plasma of venous blood. (Or 6.7 mmol/l if whole venous blood is sampled.)

- ADA: A level of glucose at or exceeding 11.1 mmol/l in the plasma of venous blood sampled at random, plus symptoms of diabetes.

  OR

  A fasting glucose level at or exceeding 7.0 mmol/l in the plasma of a venous blood sample. (Fasting is defined as no food or drink containing calories for the previous 8 to 10 hours, usually overnight.)

With both sets of criteria, repeat testing is usually carried out on consecutive days and the diagnosis is confirmed if abnormal readings continue to be obtained. A further test which may be carried out is the Oral Glucose Tolerance Test (OGTT). This has been used for some time and in revised WHO guidelines (1988) continues to be considered very important, especially in cases where the initial results are not clear cut. The OGTT has to be carried out under carefully controlled conditions and requires the person to follow a set of guidelines, summarized below.

- For at least 3 days before the test, the person must eat three meals a day containing plenty of starchy foods such as cereals, bread, pasta, and potatoes.
- An overnight fast, lasting from 10 to 16 hours, is required immediately before the test when only plain water may be drunk.
- The person must refrain from smoking and exercising immediately before and during the test.
- The test must be performed between 8 and 9 a.m. on the morning following the fast.
- A blood sample is taken to obtain a venous plasma glucose level before the test. The person is then given a flavoured drink containing 75 g of glucose dissolved in 250 ml of water, which must be consumed within 5 minutes. A second blood sample is obtained and tested after 120 minutes.
- Urine samples may occasionally require to be tested, every 30 minutes.

The OGTT has been found to be useful in identifying two intermediate states between normality and diabetes, called IMPAIRED FASTING GLUCOSE (IFG) and IMPAIRED GLUCOSE

TOLERANCE (IGT). In the OGTT, a normal result for venous plasma glucose levels is at or less than 6.0 mmol/l in the fasting state and less than 7.8 mmol/l from the second sample taken at 120 minutes. The result for diabetes is at or greater than 7.8 mmol/l during fasting and greater than 11.1 mmol/l after 120 minutes.

Blood samples taken at a doctor's surgery, clinic or hospital are normally subjected to laboratory analysis to obtain readings of blood glucose levels. People subsequently diagnosed with diabetes have to continue to monitor their blood glucose levels as part of management of the condition. There is no need to worry that this requires setting up a laboratory in the home! As described later, home testing is quite a simple procedure which does not take up a great deal of time.

Categories of Diabetes (ADA Classification, 1997)

As well as revising the diagnostic criteria for diabetes, the ADA also proposed changes of name for the two main forms of the syndrome and these terms are now in general use. Hence the former Insulin-Dependent Diabetes Mellitus or IDDM may now be called TYPE 1 DIABETES and Non-Insulin Dependent Diabetes Mellitus (NIDDM) may be termed TYPE 2 DIABETES. On a worldwide basis, Type 2 diabetes accounts for over 85 per cent of cases, although incidence varies between different ethnic groups. In the UK, more than 1.4 million people are known to have diabetes and about 80 per cent of this is Type 2.

As previously noted, diabetes is a complex series of disorders which, to a certain extent, refuses to be slotted neatly into categories. Part of the problem is that diabetic conditions may change with time. The following sections identify relevant states and syndromes, as well as the categories of diabetes that are recognized, with a brief description of each.

Impaired Fasting Glucose (IFG)

IFG is a state which is most accurately identified by means of the Oral Glucose Tolerance Test described above. It is considered to be an intermediate state, falling short of diabetes, but may be a pre-diabetic stage in some cases. It is identified when an abnormally high level of fasting glucose of 6.1 to 6.9 mmol/l is obtained from a venous plasma sample before the glucose drink is given, but a normal reading, of less than 7.8 mmol/l, exists after 120 minutes. (In normality, the fasting glucose level is at, or less than, 6.0 mmol/l.) IFG does not usually produce symptoms and the clinical implications are not, at present, fully established. A person identified with this condition may receive advice on diet, if appropriate, and further monitoring of blood glucose levels so that any changes can be identified.

Impaired Glucose Tolerance (IGT)

IGT is a second intermediate state, falling in between normality and diabetes and is one which can only be diagnosed by means of the OGGT. For IGT to exist, an abnormally high reading for fasting glucose, of 6.1 to 6.9 mmol/l, is obtained from a venous plasma sample, as in IFG. However, 120 minutes into the test, after the glucose drink has been taken, the reading remains abnormally high in the second plasma sample, at 7.8 to 11.0 mmol/l. This distinguishes IGT form both IFG and normality, in which the second reading is less than 7.8 mmol/l, and from diabetes, in which it is greater than 11.1 mmol/l. People with IGT usually do not have any symptoms but they may eventually develop Type 2 diabetes (2 to 5 per cent of those diagnosed). However, IGT can also be transitory (for example it can develop during PREGNANCY: *see* GESTATIONAL DIABETES) and some people return to normal levels of glucose tolerance with the passage of time. Defects in insulin receptors may be the cause of IGT in some cases and this may be reversible with treatment. Those with long-term, stable IGT are considered to be at greater risk both of Type 2 diabetes and also of the MACROVASCULAR COMPLICATIONS of the syndrome (such as heart disease, stroke, and conditions affecting the circulation in the legs). It is quite common for IGT (or Type 2 diabetes) to be diagnosed after a person has developed macrovascular disease, with this being the presenting condition for which the person is receiving treatment. Also, sometimes a misdiagnosis of Type 2 diabetes is made when, in fact, the person has IGT. People at a greater risk of heart disease, because of the existence of high blood pressure (hypertension), elevated levels of triglycerides, in blood plasma, high pulse rate and/or obesity, are also considered to be at high risk of IGT and/or Type 2 diabetes. In addition, the incidence of IGT is associated with ageing.

IGT and IFT are similar, and more research is being carried out to establish the exact differences and long-term implications of these two states.

Type 1 Diabetes

Type 1 diabetes (formerly Insulin-Dependent Diabetes Mellitus or IDDM) is the less common of the two main forms of diabetes and, in some ways, is easier to understand. This is because in the vast majority of cases, the diabetes arises because of a gradual and progressive autoimmune destruction of the beta islet cells of the pancreas which produce insulin. An autoimmune response can be thought of as a form of self-destruction. For some reason, the body's immune system fails to recognize some component or substance that belongs to itself and produces antibodies to attack and destroy that element, as though it were foreign or invading. In the case of Type 1 diabetes, it is the all-important insulin-producing cells that are attacked, but it takes some time for the situation to become critical. In fact, it is only after most (about 90 per cent) of the beta cells have been destroyed that the person begins to show classical symptoms of diabetes. These may include any of those described under DEFINING AND DIAGNOSING DIABETES above, but in particular, marked osmotic symptoms, weight loss and tiredness. When tests are carried out, they reveal ketonuria and significant hyperglycaemia. Usually, the symptoms are sufficiently noticeable to prompt the person to seek medical help, but this is not always the case. Unfortunately, about 5 to 10 per cent of people with Type 1 diabetes are not diagnosed until they are admitted to hospital in the emergency stage of DIABETIC KETOACIDOSIS (DKA). The key feature of Type 1 disease is that those affected need insulin replacement therapy for life in order to ensure survival.

There is a long, asymptomatic period in Type 1 diabetes (called the prodromal period) during which the beta cells are progressively being destroyed. The peak age for symptoms to appear and for diagnosis to be made is 11 to 13 years. However, this is not always the case, and mature and even elderly people are occasionally diagnosed. Initiation of insulin treatment in Type 1 diabetes quite often restores some beta cell function for a short period of time. This is known as the 'honeymoon period' and it usually lasts between six and twelve months. While it lasts, only small doses of insulin are needed and it is thought that this may extend the length of the honeymoon period itself. Unfortunately, it usually ends suddenly during a time of illness or other period of stress.

People with Type 1 diabetes have high levels of antibodies to islet cells circulating in their blood and these can be detected by laboratory analysis. Occasionally, high levels of antibodies are found in the blood of older people who were initially thought to have Type 2 diabetes, indicating that autoimmune destruction of beta cells has been taking place. These people may be designated as having Autoimmune Diabetes in Adults (LADA) to distinguish this more unusual form of Type 1 syndrome. Almost all cases of Type 1 syndrome involve autoimmune destruction of beta cells and consequent loss of insulin, as described above. However, as is so often the case in medicine, exceptions have been recorded, and in the ADA classification, this highly unusual form is designated Idiopathic Type 1 diabetes, indicating that it is of unknown origin. Affected people (who are most likely to be of African or East Asian origin) appear to have the symptoms of Type 1 syndrome and may present with ketosis, requiring emergency treatment. However, blood testing does not detect the antibodies normally associated with the disorder and the treatment needed by this unusual group may change over time. There may even be periods when their diabetes can be controlled by the ORAL ANTIDIABETIC DRUGS more appropriate to Type 2 disease.

There is a significant genetic link in the development of Type 1 diabetes and the genes involved have been identified. They are known as Class 2 major histocompatibility complex (MHC) and they are located on the short arm of chromosome 6. They are responsible for the production of Human Leukocyte Antigens (HLA), and people with genetically determined Type 1 diabetes produce certain antigens which are implicated in the autoimmune response. Many studies have been carried out to quantify the risk to an individual of developing Type 1 diabetes if he or she has a close relative already affected. Some of the most interesting studies have involved identical and non-identical twins and the approximate risks are as follows:

- mother affected: 2 to 3 per cent risk of Type 1 diabetes developing in children
- father affected: 5 to 10 per cent risk of Type 1 diabetes developing in children
- both parents affected: 30 per cent risk of development in children
- brother or sister affected: 10 per cent risk of development in siblings
- identical twin affected: 30 to 50 per cent risk of development in other twin
- non-identical twin affected: 20 per cent risk of development in other twin.

From these figures it can be seen that genetic factors at present identified do not account for all the incidence of Type 1 diabetes. It is believed that environmental factors are important, and suggested culprits include viruses (e.g. Coxsackie B4, rubella [German measles], cytomegalovirus), in utero exposure to serum albumin in cows' milk and ingestion of nitrosamines in smoked foods during infancy. It has, however, proved difficult to pinpoint environmental causes with any certainty. Their significance would seem to be confirmed by the fact that the incidence of Type 1 diabetes is rising in many countries, including the UK, where the number of children under 16 years diagnosed with the disorder doubled during the last quarter of the twentieth century.

People with Type 1 diabetes are at some risk of sudden death from severe metabolic episodes such as DKA, but in general only if specific circumstances apply or if the condition is not being managed and controlled. In the long term, there is an increased risk of diabetic complications and death from coronary heart disease or kidney failure. However, on an individual basis, there is a great deal that can be done to lower the chances of these conditions arising and to lessen the threat that they pose.

Type 2 Diabetes

More than 80 per cent of people with diabetes in Britain have this form (formerly Non-Insulin Dependent Diabetes Mellitus or NIDDM), as do the estimated 'missing million' who are currently undiagnosed. Type 2 diabetes is regarded as being a heterogeneous disorder, that is, one in which there may be two contributing defects and other associated adverse factors. One defect or adverse factor may have a relatively greater impact upon one person with the syndrome compared to another and this underlines the need for an individual approach when it comes to treatment. In contrast to Type 1 diabetes, in Type 2 disease people have a relative, rather than an absolute, loss of insulin. However, the disorder is a progressive one and in many cases the situation, both with regard to insulin secretion and the effectiveness of its action, may worsen with time. Type 2 diabetes has a long, 'silent', asymptomatic period lasting many years, and usually people are not diagnosed until they are over the age of 40 (but see below). During this time, enough insulin is produced or is effective to prevent ketosis but not enough to ensure a normal disposal of glucose. Hence there is sustained hyperglycaemia and very often the development of resultant tissue damage and diabetic COMPLICATIONS.

There are two sub-groups of Type 2 diabetes which, while they overlap with one another, tend to have somewhat different underlying causes – the two contributory defects mentioned above. People in the first sub-group, who are in the minority, are usually thin or of normal body weight. Those in this group are more likely to have a deficiency in the secretion of insulin as the underlying cause of their diabetes. In the second sub-group, comprising over 75 per cent of cases, people are likely to be overweight or obese. In those affected, INSULIN RESISTANCE is likely to be the predominant malfunction. Insulin resistance is a common feature of Type 2 diabetes and it is known that it mainly occurs at post-receptor level, affecting metabolic events that take place within cells (*see* THE BACKGROUND TO DIABETES above). However, it should be stressed that these distinctions are not necessarily clear cut and both insulin deficiency and insulin resistance can be at work in either sub-group of Type 2 diabetes.

The significance of obesity and the importance of weight control are discussed in a later chapter of this book. However, there is universal agreement among medical experts that the rising tide of obesity among people in Western countries is closely linked with an escalating incidence of Type 2 diabetes that is reaching epidemic proportions. Of particular concern is the fact that Type 2 syndrome has recently been identified in obese teenagers, both in the USA and in Britain. It is feared that since many more children are now significantly overweight or obese than was the case a generation ago, cases of early Type 2 diabetes will become more common. Indeed, one study in Plymouth showed that 26 per cent of 5-year-old girls surveyed were not only overweight but were exhibiting early signs of resistance to insulin.

People least likely to be affected are those living in countries where a traditional lifestyle and diet are followed. At greatest risk are those who have rapidly changed from eating a traditional diet to a Western one and some racial groups also appear to be particularly vulnerable (e.g. South Asians living in Britain). There is a strong genetic/inheritance link in the development of Type 2 diabetes but less is known about the genes involved. The familial pattern is as follows:

- one parent affected: 15 to 40 per cent risk of Type 2 diabetes in offspring and higher if mother is the diabetic parent
- both parents affected: 50 to 75 per cent risk of Type 2 diabetes in offspring
- identical twin affected: 90 per cent risk of development of Type 2 diabetes in other twin.

Environmental factors, especially the development of obesity coupled with a lack of exercise, greatly increase the chances of developing Type 2 diabetes. Smoking is another known hazard. Other risk factors include being of low birth weight due to inadequate foetal nutrition during development, especially if the person becomes overweight in adult life. Certain endocrine (hormonal) disorders, drug treatments, a previous history of glucose intolerance and/

or INSULIN RESISTANCE, and, in females, GESTATIONAL DIABETES are other pre-disposing factors. As previously mentioned, signs and symptoms for Type 2 diabetes are highly variable, depending upon the stage of progression of the disorder and the extent of insulin loss. When present, they usually include osmotic symptoms and tiredness, vision disturbance and possibly, recurrent infections. Weight loss and ketonuria are absent and the person is usually middle aged or elderly. Diabetic COMPLICATIONS are quite commonly present at diagnosis, reflecting the fact that the syndrome is often not identified until quite a late stage, when tissue damage has already taken place.

Other Specific Forms of Diabetes Mellitus

Genetic Defects Affecting Pancreatic Beta Cells, e.g. Maturity Onset Diabetes of the Young (MODY)
This is an unusual form of diabetes, which has been the subject of considerable research in recent years. Although it superficially resembles Type 2 diabetes, there are a number of important differences. MODY appears in childhood or young adulthood, before the age of 25 years, and in most cases at least one or even two other members of the immediate family are affected. It has an entirely genetic origin and the defects (or mutations) in the genes involved have been identified. Environmental factors do not contribute to MODY and those affected are of normal weight and rarely obese. Five sub-groups of MODY have been identified (MODY 1, 2, 3, 4, 5 – depending upon the precise mutations in the genes involved) which produce diabetes of varying degrees of severity. Hence treatment also varies accordingly, with one form usually managed by

diet alone while others require drug or insulin therapy. The risk of complications likewise varies between the different forms of MODY. In one in five families affected by this syndrome, the genetic defect involved is not one that has been previously identified. Hence it is likely that further sub-groups of MODY will emerge in the future when further mutations are identified. The pattern of inheritance involved in MODY is called 'autosomal dominance' and there is a 50 per cent risk of diabetes in the child of an affected parent. It has been suggested that genetic screening of the offspring of a MODY parent might be helpful but there is also concern that this might raise more problems than it solves. Although 'at risk' children with the genetic defect for MODY can be identified, it is far from certain that any preventive treatment that may be attempted will be effective.

Genetic Defects in Insulin Action, e.g.'Leprechaunism' and Rabson-Mendenhall Syndrome

There are a number of rare, genetic abnormalities affecting the insulin receptors, resulting in severe disruption of their structure and function. Severe insulin resistance and diabetes are characteristic of these syndromes, along with various other metabolic features.

Diseases of the Exocrine Pancreas, e.g. Pancreatitis, Cystic Fibrosis, Haemochromatosis

The pancreas is vulnerable to a number of conditions and disorders which, if severe, may cause secondary diabetes. *Pancreatitis* (inflammation of the pancreas) may be acute (and usually transient), or chronic and long-lasting (often caused by alcoholism). People with the chronic condition are at risk of diabetes, as are those with cancer of the pancreas and patients who have undergone surgical removal (pancreatectomy) of the whole or part of the gland as a method of treatment. Cystic fibrosis is a condition that affects all the glands of the body, including the pancreas. Improved treatment for sufferers and increased survival times mean that diabetes is a common complication, usually appearing in the teenage years or young adulthood and eventually requiring insulin therapy. Haemochromatosis is a rare metabolic, genetic disorder which is characterized by iron being deposited in various organs, including the liver and pancreas. Diabetes requiring insulin treatment develops in about half of those affected. It is sometimes called 'bronzed diabetes' due to an unusual pigmentation of the skin which is a feature of haemochromatosis. The disorder causes a number of serious complications, of which diabetes is only one and sufferers require intensive treatment.

Diabetes that Develops as a Feature of Endocrinopathies

Endocrinopathies (diseases due to disorders of the *endocrine glands*) and in particular autoimmune conditions, such as *Graves' disease*, acromegaly, and *Cushings syndrome*, primarily affect hormone-secreting glands, causing hormone imbalances which affect the production and action of insulin. It has also been found that people with Type 1 diabetes run an increased risk of developing other autoimmune disorders. People suffering from these conditions are likewise at greater risk of developing diabetes which may require insulin treatment or INSULIN RESISTANCE or IMPAIRED GLUCOSE TOLERANCE.

Some other autoimmune disorders, e.g. *Addison's disease*, primary hypothyroidism and so-called Stiff Man syndrome, are associated with an increased sensitivity to insulin and hence HYPOGLYCAEMIA. People with Type 1 diabetes run an increased risk of developing these types of disorders.

Coeliac disease or gluten enteropathy is another autoimmune condition with some similarities to diabetes. It is a wasting disease in which the intestines are unable to absorb fat. There may be hypoglycaemia caused by malabsorption and the symptoms are caused by an intolerance to the protein, gluten, found in wheat and rye flour, which damages the lining of the intestines. It is treated by a strict and lifelong adherence to a gluten-free diet but some people also have an additional need for insulin therapy.

Diabetes Caused by Drugs or Chemicals, e.g. Coticosteroids, Thiazide Diuretics and Beta-blockers

Quite a number of drug treatments are associated with the development of glucose intolerance, insulin resistance or diabetes. Also, when these drugs are taken by people with existing diabetes, they may lead to a lowering of glycaemic control so that someone with Type 2 syndrome that had been managed with tablets may then require insulin. It may be that some patients are in a higher risk group for glucose intolerance, insulin resistance or diabetes, or are undiagnosed for these conditions at the start of drug treatment. Many of the drugs are used to treat serious conditions with a known link to diabetes such as hormonal disorders, HYPERTENSION and heart and circulatory disease.

Diabetes Caused by Infections, e.g. Congenital German Measles (Rubella)

Various viral infections have been implicated in the development of Type 1 diabetes. Infection of a developing foetus with rubella leads to a 20 to 40 per cent risk of autoimmune diabetes in the child.

Uncommon Forms of Immune-mediated Diabetes

This is a group of rare disorders, such as Stiff Man syndrome, which are associated with the development of diabetes.

Other Genetic Syndromes which may confer a Greater Risk of Diabetes

A number of inherited, chromosomal abnormalities carry an increased risk of diabetes. Their number include *Down's syndrome, Turner's syndrome, Klinefelter's syndrome, Friedreich's ataxia*, neonatal diabetes, and mitochondrial syndromes passed through the maternal line.

Gestational Diabetes Mellitus: Diabetes First Diagnosed in Pregnancy

This is regarded as a special category which includes IMPAIRED GLUCOSE TOLERANCE and transient diabetes, both precipitated and diagnosed in pregnancy but resolving after the birth, and diabetes that has been pre-existing but first comes to light during pregnancy. While transient diabetes and IGT usually disappear after delivery, affected women have a greater risk of eventually developing Type 2 diabetes. Women with pre-existing but formerly unsuspected diabetes are usually older mothers who are overweight or obese, and in almost all cases they are affected by Type 2 syndrome. These women continue to need treatment for their diabetes following delivery. A small number of, usually

young, women diagnosed with gestational diabetes are dis-
covered to have Type 1 syndrome. It is thought that the
metabolic changes that occur during pregnancy (which
for all women are pro-diabetic) may exacerbate or at least
reveal the existence of diabetes that had previously not
reached a stage of producing symptoms.

The incidence of gestational diabetes varies between
different populations and racial groups. Southern Asian
women are affected at twice the rate (4 to 5 per cent) of
white Europeans (1 to 2 per cent). Women belonging to
some racial groups (e.g. Latin Americans) who develop gestational diabetes that initially resolves, nevertheless are at
greater risk of a fairly rapid development of Type 2 diabetes.

The special care of pregnant women with diabetes is
discussed in Chapter 10. The more unusual categories of
(secondary) diabetes described above have been included
as a matter of interest and information. Treatment of these
conditions may require a multi-targeted approach of which
diabetes control may be only one aspect. The information
in the remaining chapters of this book mostly relate to the
common forms of diabetes, Type 1 and Type 2, that are also
the most familiar.

Conditions that Contribute to and are Closely Related to Diabetes

The conditions described below are often a component of
diabetes (especially of Type 2 syndrome) and may themselves contribute to the existence of the condition.

Insulin Resistance

We have already seen that resistance to the effects of insulin,
which usually appears to act at the level beyond the receptor

sites, is of major significance in Type 2 diabetes. Insulin resistance is defined as a reduced response or sensitivity to a physiological amount of insulin (i.e. a quantity which would be expected to have an identifiable effect). Its existence is suspected when a test of a venous blood plasma sample after a fast reveals an abnormally high level of insulin (hyperinsulinaemia) in the presence of a normal or raised level of blood glucose. Sensitivity to insulin can be determined using a laboratory technique called the hyperinsulinaemic glucose clamp. A certain quantity of insulin is infused and at the same time, dextrose (a form of sugar) is also given. The more sugar that is required to maintain a normal blood glucose level during the period of elevated insulin caused by the infusion, the greater the person's sensitivity to insulin. Studies suggest that there is considerable variation in the degree of insulin sensitivity in apparently healthy people, and insulin resistance as such does not cause any symptoms. Indeed, about one quarter of those surveyed have degrees of insulin resistance comparable with those in people diagnosed with glucose intolerance or Type 2 diabetes. It is known that sustained hyperinsulinaemia, as occurs in insulin resistance, increases the risk of the development of cardiovascular complications. Insulin resistance naturally increases during puberty and pregnancy, but in normal health this is compensated for by an increased production of insulin. Sensitivity returns to normal once these states are past. Insulin resistance can also be caused by drugs and is also much more likely to occur in people who are obese, especially in those who have upper body, abdominal fat deposits. This type of obesity is similarly closely linked with the incidence of Type 2 diabetes. It is further believed that lack of exercise and cigarette smoking may make insulin resistance worse in some cases.

Insulin Resistance Syndrome

This syndrome was first described in 1988 and has a number of alternative names (Reaven's syndrome, metabolic syndrome, syndrome X). It has several components and usually more than one is present in those affected. The key features, identified in 1988, are:

- glucose intolerance or Type 2 diabetes
- decreased level/rate of glucose disposal by insulin
- hyperinsulinaemia-
- essential hypertension (high blood pressure)
- low plasma levels of HDL lipoproteins
- hypertriglyceridaemia (high levels of triglyceride fats in the blood).

Since 1988, other factors have been added which were felt to be important, including abdominal obesity and impaired fibrinolysis – a process that normally takes place in the blood by means of which minute blood clots are broken down. Insulin resistance syndrome confers a much greater risk of *atherosclerosis* or furring of the arteries and coronary heart disease. People with Type 2 diabetes or IMPAIRED GLUCOSE TOLERANCE quite often show features of the syndrome (such as HYPERTENSION). It is necessary to treat these conditions, alongside diabetes, when they are present in order to reduce the risk of cardiovascular disease.

Polycystic Ovary Syndrome and Insulin Resistance

In women, the relatively common condition called polycystic ovary syndrome, in which the follicles of the ovaries fail to produce eggs to maturity and develop multiple small cysts, may in some cases be linked with insulin resistance, in some cases. Polycystic ovary syndrome is caused by a hormonal imbalance which results in a greater than normal availability of male sex hormones (*androgens*, mainly *testosterone*) which may stimulate a masculine pattern of hair growth in some women. The ovaries normally produce minute quantities of androgens which are 'mopped up' by proteins called *globulins*. It is thought that hyperinsulinaemia in insulin resistance may stimulate the production of testosterone by the ovaries and also inhibit the production of globulin. This allows more testosterone to be available, producing the symptoms of polycystic ovary syndrome. It has been found that affected women may have a greater susceptibility to Type 2 diabetes. Also, women affected by GESTATIONAL DIABETES run a greater risk of developing polycystic ovary syndrome.

Abdominal (or Visceral) Obesity

As has been noted, there is a close connection between obesity and Type 2 diabetes and it is thought that upper body or abdominal fat may be particularly important. However, although men are more likely to show this pattern of fat distribution than women (who more frequently lay down fat below the waist), there is no apparent sex difference in the incidence of Type 2 diabetes. The main function of abdominal adipocytes (fat cells) is to store triglycerides as an energy reserve in times of need. (*See* THE BACKGROUND TO DIABETES above.) These fat cells have been shown to have a different metabolic activity compared to other fat cells elsewhere, particularly with regard to their sensitivity to certain hormones. They have been found to be more resistant to insulin but show greater sensitivity to catecholamines (counter-regulatory hormones) which act in opposition to insulin. Hence it is felt by some experts that abdominal obesity promotes the type of insulin resistance that is often a feature of Type 2 diabetes, although it is probably only one contributory factor and may not be enough to cause diabetes in itself.

Hypertension

High blood pressure can occur on its own but it is often a feature of Type 2 diabetes and the insulin resistance syndrome. Less commonly, it may also be associated with Type 1 syndrome as well. It is believed that the physiological and metabolic consequences of insulin resistance and Type 2 diabetes promote the development of hypertension and that the two are closely linked (*see* Chapter 9).

2

INITIAL DIAGNOSIS AND EARLY CARE

Diagnosis and Referral

In the UK, it is usually the general practitioner who initially suspects, identifies or diagnoses diabetes. As noted earlier, the patient may have come to see the doctor with marked symptoms that indicate the condition. However, it is quite common for diabetes to come to light incidentally, during the course of some other medical examination or check-up. Usually, a urine sample will have been tested (by means of a stick that changes colour in the presence of glucose) and a positive result will have prompted the doctor to look for other signs of diabetes. *Glycosuria* is not in itself diagnostic of diabetes, and, even more important, its absence at a particular moment does not necessarily mean that there is no diabetes. Several factors can influence glycosuria, including certain drug treatments, fluid intake and urine concentration and, most significantly, the person's renal threshold for glucose. The renal threshold is the level or concentration at which glucose is reabsorbed into the body during the process of filtration in the kidneys. Those with a low renal threshold, notably children in normal health, are hence much more likely to show glycosuria. Conversely, elderly people are far more likely to have a high renal threshold and glycosuria may be absent even in the presence of diabetes. This is why it is usual for a finger prick test for blood glucose (similar to that used for self-monitoring in established diabetes) to be carried out. If results indicate the likelihood of diabetes, a telephone referral is made to the local diabetes clinic which often operates from the nearest hospital. If the situation is urgent – the person has serious osmotic symptoms or ketonuria, feels ill, or is judged to be at risk of ACUTE METABOLIC COMPLICATIONS – arrangements are made for emergency admittance to hospital. If the person is not at risk, the appointment to attend the diabetes clinic will be as soon as possible. Those with Type 1 diabetes have the greatest priority and will usually be seen immediately.

Staff at a typical hospital-based diabetes clinic usually include the following:

• consultant diabetologist (a specialist in diabetes)
• specialist diabetes nurses (Specialist nurses are highly trained in all aspects of diabetes care including patient education, administering and monitoring of treatment and alteration of doses, management of all aspects of diabetes and its complications on a long-term basis, and referral to specialists when required. The nurse is the person with whom the patient has most contact and he or she may also undertake home visits and community-based care.)
• dietitian
• podiatrist (specialist in foot care).

Diabetic patients may also require the help of other specialists from time to time, especially in connection with the complications of their condition. These may include:

• cardiologist (heart specialist)
• vascular surgeon (specialist in diseased and damaged blood vessels)

- nephrologist (specialist in kidney disease)
- ophthalmologist (eye specialist).

Living with diabetes can have a considerable PSYCHO-LOGICAL impact and there is a higher than normal risk of depression. Some people benefit from psychological counselling, and staff at the diabetes clinic are able to make referrals to a psychologist/psychotherapist, when this is considered to be helpful or necessary (*see* Chapter 11, PSYCHOLOGICAL ASPECTS OF DIABETES).

Initial Consultation

The initial consultation at the clinic usually requires more time than is necessary for follow-up appointments. Members of the clinical team need to acquire and impart a lot of information and set aside time for discussion. It is necessary to obtain as full a picture as possible, not only of the person's medical history but of their family and social background, work, and lifestyle as well. A thorough physical examination is required. Plenty of time is allowed for discussion and answering the inevitable questions that arise, the whole aim being to allay anxiety and to establish the basis of a good relationship for the future. Questions and subjects for discussion include:

- symptoms, if present; implications of blood glucose levels; explanation of diabetes
- diet and lifestyle; alcohol consumption; smoking; current exercise pattern; occupation and nature of work duties; drug use, prescription or otherwise
- family history of diabetes, if any
- for women, obstetric history; GESTATIONAL DIABETES; birth weights of children; menstrual history
- existing medical conditions and their treatment

- physical examination, which will include:
- height and weight (calculation of body/mass index which is used to determine the presence of obesity)
- blood pressure, recorded both lying down and standing up
- signs/symptoms of diabetic COMPLICATIONS, e.g. examination of feet and eyes. (People with Type 2 diabetes are much more likely to have complications at the time of diagnosis.)

Although it is often possible to confirm the category of diabetes during the course of the consultation, this is not always straightforward. As has been seen, diabetes is a condition that crosses boundaries and can throw up exceptions to the rule. From the clinical point of view, the most important decision to be made is to determine the appropriate course of action and in particular whether the person requires insulin therapy straight away. Patients with Type 1 diabetes, which, by definition, is insulin-dependent, will almost certainly have an immediate need for insulin. Occasionally, however, results are equivocal, perhaps because the diabetes has been detected early while the person is still producing some insulin and classical symptoms are not present. Such a person may well be started on ORAL ANTIDIABETIC DRUGS to begin with but will eventually require insulin. Conversely, a person with Type 2 diabetes may have blood results and symptoms indicating the need for initial insulin treatment, particularly if he or she has been suffering from a bout of illness. Later, it may be possible for the diabetes to be managed by a combination of diet control and medication.

Based on all their findings and clinical evaluation, the diabetes team will work out an initial treatment programme with the co-operation of the person concerned, taking into account that this may require some adjustment at a later date. The aims of treatment are:

- to relieve symptoms of diabetes, if present
- to prevent (or lessen the progression of) diabetic complications and to relieve their symptoms
- to teach the person with Type 1 diabetes how to recognize and deal with HYPOGLYCAEMIA
- in the longer term, to help the person to lead a long, full and active life
- to try and achieve this with the minimum possible disruption to normal life.

Understanding and Managing Diabetes

Successful treatment and management of diabetes very much depend upon the motivation and positive engagement of the affected person. There is a considerable element of self-management involved and so the person with diabetes needs to acquire knowledge about the condition and to understand why he or she is advised to follow a certain course of action. It is a very good idea for the person's family to be involved as well, and education about all aspects of the condition is a very important part of the work of the diabetes clinical care team. Usually, the diabetic person will be asked to attend the first examination/ interview in the company of a close family member so that the process of education can begin straight away. There are very many aspects to this but the most important is that it should be tailored to the individual needs of the person concerned. It is an ongoing process and the requirements may change over time. Many clinics offer group sessions after the initial interview, covering everyday aspects of LIVING WITH DIABETES and allowing plenty of time for discussion. These can be very helpful, allowing new friendships to be made and experiences to be shared in an informal and enjoyable way. There are a variety of educational materials available dealing with different aspects of diabetes, including leaflets, books and videos, which are a helpful source of information that can be referred to at home.

During the initial interview, general educational aims will include:

- establishing a good relationship or partnership with the person and listening to his or her views
- exploring the person's current beliefs about diabetes and other health issues with a view to correcting any that are inaccurate
- attempting to get to know the whole person by talking about family, work responsibilities, cultural and religious beliefs etc., all of which may affect his or her ability to manage diabetes
- explaining clearly the nature of diabetes and the reasons behind a proposed programme of treatment which is likely to include some of the following: diet and weight control, lifestyle changes, exercise, and drug or insulin treatment
- setting realistic goals, worked out in partnership, which the person feels able to achieve
- explaining and demonstrating all aspects of management and treatment, probably including HOME BLOOD GLUCOSE MONITORING, HOME URINE TESTING, when to take tablets and the effects that they will have, when and how to self-inject insulin and the type and nature of the insulin being

used. All this will be worked out so that it can fit in with the person's usual daily routine.

- ensuring that the person understands the importance of attending subsequent appointments and how to get in touch quickly with the diabetes care team, should the need arise
- asking the person how he or she feels about the diagnosis of diabetes in order to assess the person's state of mind and giving reassurance, when necessary.

PSYCHOLOGICAL factors have a major impact on the treatment and management of diabetes. The person may be in a state of shock on receiving the diagnosis and may be finding it hard to absorb the information that is being given. It is very important that this should be recognized and that the person is dealt with sensitively and feels supported by the clinical team. Plenty of time may be needed to discuss the person's fears and to endeavour to build his or her self-confidence and belief in the ability to cope. Hence the amount of information (education) given in the first instance may need to be limited to that which is strictly necessary and the person may possibly be referred for further counselling or psychological care.

3

DIETARY AND DRUG TREATMENT

Type 1 diabetes is treated by means of DIETARY MODIFICA-TION or NUTRITION THERAPY and INSULIN TREATMENT. Type 2 diabetes is treated by means of dietary modification alone, dietary modification and drug therapy (using ORAL ANTIDIABETIC DRUGS), dietary modification with combined insulin and drug therapy, or dietary modification and insulin therapy. In the latter case, the diabetes is said to be insulin-treated Type 2 diabetes, as distinct from insulin-dependent Type 1 diabetes. Taking regular EXERCISE, although not a treatment method itself, has an important part to play in the overall management of diabetes. This chapter deals with treatment by means of diet and drugs (with a short section on surgical treatment for rare and advanced conditions), and insulin treatment is discussed in Chapter 4.

Dietary Modification or Nutrition Therapy

Dietary modification forms an important part of the treatment and management of all types of diabetes. In Type 2 diabetes, it is almost always connected with the need to lose weight since the majority of people with this syndrome (75 per cent) are overweight or obese. Hence, even though there may be slightly different underlying reasons, the dietary advice for all forms of diabetes is essentially the same. Also, a good diet for people with diabetes conforms entirely to current nutritional guidelines on healthy eating for the population as a whole. It may be quite helpful for people newly diagnosed with diabetes to feel that they need to follow a 'healthy eating' plan rather than a 'diabetic diet' and that this plan is good for everyone else too! In fact, the whole concept of the diabetic diet is now considered to be outmoded as is any need for special 'diabetic foods'. These are still available, mainly from chemists and pharmacies, but they are both expensive and unnecessary since the person with diabetes can fulfil all nutritional requirements from ordinary foods.

The general aims behind dietary modification in diabetes can be summarized as follows:

- to improve carbohydrate and fat metabolism in order to help maintain blood glucose levels within an acceptable range
- to achieve an appropriate body weight (according to age, state of health etc.). This, in itself, very often improves glucose control in Type 2 diabetes
- to reduce the occurrence of HYPOGLYCAEMIA (in those being treated with insulin or SULPHONYLUREAS)
- to help prevent or slow down the development of diabetic COMPLICATIONS
- to reduce the risks of circulatory disease and HYPERTENSION (through weight control, often combined with physical exercise).

Each newly diagnosed person will have an interview with a dietitian so that his or her individual requirements can be assessed. The person's current eating habits and lifestyle will be discussed in detail and suggestions made for easily incorporated adjustments which will improve diabetes. If the person needs to lose weight, sensible ways of achieving this will be looked into and included in the dietary plan. Often, a person has become overweight in the first place because of an over-reliance on foods high in (saturated) fats and sugar. Changing to a more healthy pattern of eating, especially when combined with an increased amount of exercise, will usually produce a sustained, gradual loss of weight without the person needing to go hungry. In fact, the whole aim of nutrition therapy in diabetes is to produce a pattern of eating which the person feels readily able to adopt and to set a realistic and achievable weight-loss target, if appropriate. Severe calorie-restriction diets, reliance on drugs, or extreme surgical measures normally have no place in this, except perhaps in very rare circumstances.

Dietary Advice

In broad terms, dietary advice for a person newly diagnosed with diabetes is likely to include the following.

- Eat three, well-spaced meals a day, preferably at the same, regular times and do not miss meals. This is especially important for people being treated with insulin or the category of ORAL ANTIDIABETIC DRUGS known as SULPHONYLUREAS. These people are also likely to need additional snacks, for example, just before bedtime, to reduce the risk of HYPOGLYCAEMIA.

- Cut down on sugar and avoid obviously sugary foods. Modern advice is that there is no need to avoid sugar completely, as this is very difficult anyway, but to switch to low-sugar or sugar-free varieties of manufactured foods and drinks. Sweeteners should be used in coffee, tea or home-prepared foods such as stewed fruit, custard etc. Many home-baking recipes can be adapted to contain less sugar (and fat) so that favourite foods can still be enjoyed in moderation. Diabetes UK produces a helpful booklet containing useful tips and recipes. Small quantities of sweets or chocolate are usually permissible, as long as they are only eaten sparingly and after a high carbohydrate meal. People with Type 1 diabetes occasionally require some form of sugar (often a sweet drink, jam, honey or glucose sweets), to treat a HYPOGLYCAEMIC attack or 'hypo'.

- Eat more foods containing starch and fibre. Starch is a complex carbohydrate which takes a longer time to be digested and absorbed into the bloodstream as glucose. This is particularly helpful in diabetes as it avoids the 'peaking' of blood glucose levels that tends to occur when simple carbohydrates such as sugar are eaten. Eating starch, especially when combined with fibre, slows digestion and provides a steady and sustained supply of energy which is particularly helpful in diabetes, especially for those receiving insulin. Good sources of starch include cereals, bread, pasta, potatoes, pulses etc., and it is recommended that these foods should provide 55 per cent of total calories for those with diabetes. This is only slightly higher than the advised level for the population as a whole which is 50 per cent. Many high-starch foods are also good sources of fibre and this is particularly true of wholemeal varieties of the above and, for example, potatoes with their skins left on. A diet containing plenty of fibre is healthy for everyone and is now considered to be protective against diseases of the lower bowel, including cancer. High fibre foods are filling without being fattening and are an ideal choice for those who need to lose weight. Fibre slows down both eating and the digestive process, encouraging a person to eat only what they need and enabling a sustained absorption of glucose into the blood, which is particularly helpful in diabetes. There are two forms of fibre, insoluble and soluble. Insoluble fibre includes wheat and cereal bran, and cellulose found in green vegetables. The best way of incorporating more of this into the diet is to choose wholemeal/wholegrain varieties of staple foods and to try and eat more vegetables. Soluble fibre is found in oats, fruit, peas, beans, lentils and other pulses. It has been shown to lower blood cholesterol and triglyceride levels and improve blood glucose profiles. This in turn, reduces the risk of atherosclerosis and consequent heart and circulatory disease, which is especially important in diabetes.

- Eat more fresh fruit, vegetables and salad. It is recommended that everyone should eat at least five portions of fresh fruit and vegetables each day (not including potatoes) and these foods are especially important in diabetes. They not only supply carbohydrate and soluble fibre but vitamins, minerals and antioxidants which are beneficial for health and may help to protect against heart and circulatory disease and some cancers. Fruit is an ideal snack for a person with diabetes and can be helpful in a weight-loss programme as it is low in fat and calories. Although it contains some sugar (in the form of fructose), fruit has a small effect overall on levels of blood glucose. For those with Type 1 diabetes, it can be eaten as a replacement for other forms of carbohydrate.

- Change to a low-fat (but not a no-fat) diet and in particular, cut down on consumption of saturated fats. Saturated fats are the type found in red meat, butter, full-fat milk, cheese and cream and some other dairy products and are 'hidden' in many manufactured foods such as meat pies, sausages, biscuits, cakes etc. Excess consumption of saturated fats in Western diets is held to be responsible for many cases of heart and circulatory disease. Also, it is heavily implicated in the development of obesity and its consequences, which may include the development of insulin resistance and Type 2 diabetes. Polyunsaturated or monounsaturated fats such as those found in vegetable oils (sunflower, olive, safflower, soya etc.) and margarines should be eaten sparingly as a substitute for saturated fats. For those with diabetes, it is recommended that no more than 35 per cent of total daily calories should be derived from fats, with a preferred level at about 30 per cent. Saturated fat consumption should be no greater than 10 per cent of the total with the remainder being poly- or monounsaturated fats. Oily fish, which are a source of polyunsaturated fats, contain omega-3 fish oils which have been shown to be protective against heart and circulatory disease and these should be eaten regularly. All these recommendations are equally applicable to people who are not affected by diabetes.
- In order to reduce overall fat intake and to choose the 'right' sort of fat, the following guidelines may be given.
  - Change to semi-skimmed or skimmed milk.
  - Use low-fat spreads sparingly instead of full-fat, hard margarine or butter.
  - Do not fry or roast food – grill, bake, boil, steam or

microwave it instead. Stir-frying, with just a smear of oil, is a good method too.

○ Cut off all visible fat from meat before cooking and choose lean varieties. Eat smaller portions, less frequently and choose lean chicken or turkey (the white meat is lower in fat), fish, shellfish or pulses as an alternative to red meat.

○ Cut right down on consumption of manufactured high-fat foods such as pies, sausages, biscuits, cakes and chocolate. Eat less pastry.

○ There are many fat-reduced types of popular cheeses such as cheddar, now available. Change to these and eat them sparingly. Try low fat varieties such as cottage cheese or fat-reduced soft cheese for a change.

○ Bulk out stews, casseroles etc. with vegetables and pulses and reduce the amount of meat used. Try soya or quorn mince as a substitute for beef mince in bolognese etc.

• For most people with diabetes, it is recommended that no more than 15 per cent of the total daily intake of calories should be derived from protein. Protein is found both in foods of animal origin (meat, fish, poultry, eggs, cheese etc.) and in vegetable-based ones (such as pulses, nuts, wholegrains, seeds). Small portions of protein-rich foods should be eaten regularly by people with diabetes, as part of a balanced diet. Fish, including oily fish, is a valuable source of animal protein as well as having other beneficial properties. However, some people, especially those with Type 1 syndrome, may be recommended to follow a protein-restricted diet, obtaining no more than 12 per cent of daily total calories from protein-rich foods. This particularly applies to those with early DIABETIC NEPHROPATHY (kidney disease, *see* Chapter 8), for whom there is some evidence that restriction of protein intake may slow progression of the condition. For people with advanced NEPH-ROPATHY, more severe protein restriction may be needed, under medical supervision.

- Restrict alcohol consumption. Evidence suggests that for most people with diabetes (especially for those with Type 2 syndrome), moderate consumption of alcohol within recommended safe limits may be beneficial. Modest drinking is associated with a lowered risk of coronary heart disease and atherosclerosis, a lower level of circulating insulin, a higher level of helpful HDL cholesterol and a reduction in blood-clotting tendency. There may be a decreased risk of developing Type 2 diabetes among those who drink moderately. A safe and health-enhancing level of alcohol consumption has been set at:
  - no more than 30 g or 3 units each day for men
  - no more than 20 g or 2 units each day for women. (A unit is equivalent to 375 ml or half a pint of beer, 120 ml or one small glass of wine or 44 ml or a single pub measure of spirits.)

It is further recommended that there should be one or two alcohol-free days each week and that total weekly consumption should not exceed 21 units for men and 14 units for women. Drinking alcohol at a greater level than this not only wipes out all the potential benefits but also has proven detrimental effects upon health. People with diabetes, especially those who are at risk of HYPOGLYCAEMIA, have to be particularly careful with alcohol. Most alcoholic drinks have a high sugar/calorie content and hence are not helpful for those trying to lose weight. It is sensible to avoid alcoholic drinks with a high sugar content such as sweet wines, sherries and liqueurs.

However, the main risk is that of HYPOGLYCAEMIA, in those who are receiving treatment with SULPHONYLUREAS or insulin, which can occur many hours after the alcohol has been consumed and even the next day, in some cases. In susceptible people, hypoglycaemia can occur even when they have consumed a modest amount of alcohol, which would not normally be expected to cause problems or intoxication. A further risk for diabetic people is that symptoms of hypoglycaemia can all too easily be mistaken for drunkenness and appropriate help may not be forthcoming. The reason why alcohol poses particular problems lies with metabolic processes in the liver. Metabolism of alcohol inhibits gluconeogenesis (*see* Chapter 1, THE BACKGROUND TO DIABETES) which would normally produce glucose, and risks are particularly high after a fast. In order to lessen the chance of alcohol-related hypoglycaemia, people at risk are given the following advice.

○ Limit alcohol consumption and only drink while eating a high-carbohydrate containing meal.
○ Never drink alcohol on an empty stomach.
○ Avoid low-calorie drinks which are often higher in alcohol.
○ Be alert to the risk of NOCTURNAL HYPOGLYCAEMIA or hypoglycaemia which can occur the following day. A high fibre, carbohydrate snack should be eaten before going to bed and you may need to ADJUST THE INSULIN DOSE. Ask your clinical diabetes team for advice.

◦ Alert family and friends to the risk and carry diabetes identification.

Some people with particular COMPLICATIONS, such as elevated triglyceride levels in the blood (hypertriglyceridaemia), DIABETIC NEUROPATHY and persistent HYPERTENSION are advised to avoid alcohol altogether.

- Cut down on salt. Most people eat far more salt than they need and this is potentially harmful to health and puts a strain on the kidneys. Excess salt intake may contribute to HYPERTENSION and heart and circulatory disorders, both of which pose a particular threat to people with diabetes. This is because many of those with Type 2 diabetes already have high blood pressure to some degree and cutting down on salt, along with losing weight if obese, are measures that can help. There are several fairly simple ways to reduce salt intake.

  ◦ Eat fewer manufactured foods, which often have a high salt content. Check labels carefully.
  ◦ In home cooking, try flavouring foods with herbs and spices and use little or no salt.
  ◦ Do not add salt at the table.
  ◦ Do not use potassium salt substitutes without first obtaining medical advice.

Many people with Type 2 diabetes will be treated by dietary modification alone for a period of three months. For the majority, this involves following a diet aimed at sustained, steady weight loss combined with increased physical exercise and other lifestyle changes such as stopping smoking. Unfortunately, in the longer term, nutrition therapy alone is successful only for a minority of people with the condition. At any particular time, it is estimated that 20 per cent of people with Type 2 diabetes are being treated by nutrition therapy alone, 50 per cent with tablets and the remaining 30 per cent with insulin. Some newly diagnosed people may require tablets or insulin from the start. This is more likely to be the case for people of normal weight who are already eating a healthy diet. Nutrition therapy remains an excellent option for those who are overweight or obese, whether they require additional treatment or not, since losing weight is associated with a lowering of blood glucose and circulating lipid (fat) levels. Also, there may be a beneficial lowering of high blood pressure and a reduction in the risks of heart and circulatory disease.

Oral Antidiabetic Drugs

As mentioned above, half of those with Type 2 diabetes are treated with oral antidiabetic drugs in combination with nutrition therapy. The drugs used to treat diabetes can be classified according to their mode of action as

- hypoglycaemic agents, i.e. those which act to lower blood glucose levels
- anti-hyperglycaemic agents, i.e. those which act to prevent blood glucose levels from rising.

There are four groups of oral antidiabetic drugs, which can be classified as shown below.

Hypoglycaemic drugs	Anti-hyperglycaemic drugs
sulphonylureas	biguanides (metformin)
meglitinides (repaglinide)	alpha-glucosidase inhibitors (acarbose)

The anti-hyperglycaemic drugs, when used as the only treatment, do not cause HYPOGLYCAEMIA. The choice of anti-diabetic drug is initially made by careful assessment of all the individual factors relevant to the person's condition. These may include presence or absence of osmotic symptoms, blood glucose levels and glycaemic control, presence or absence of diabetic COMPLICATIONS, previous response to nutrition therapy, body weight, and other medication being taken. A drug belonging to one group may be used at first as monotherapy (i.e. the only one prescribed) but it may later prove necessary to add another drug from a different group. It is also necessary to choose the most appropriate drug from within the group as each has somewhat different properties. However, oral antidiabetic drugs are not prescribed for pregnant women or nursing mothers who are treated with insulin.

Sulphonylureas
Sulphonylureas work by increasing the sensitivity of the beta islet cells of the pancreas to glucose so that they release more insulin in response to the presence of a particular level of blood glucose. They also stimulate the uptake of glucose from the blood by peripheral and muscle tissues and they lower hepatic (liver) production of glucose. Sulphonylureas can only work in people who still have some operational beta cells that are able to produce insulin. There are a number of drugs within the group (*see* below) which act metabolically in slightly different ways. One of the principal differences between them is the length of time for which they remain detectable in blood plasma (known as the half-life of the drug), which is a reflection of the length of time for which they remain active. In general,

those with a longer half-life pose a greater threat of a more prolonged HYPOGLYCAEMIA, which is the most severe potential side-effect of these drugs and which in rare cases can cause serious neurological damage or death. All the sulphonylureas remain active, that is, produce glucose-lowering effects, for a longer period than their half-life, although there are differences between them. Some of this group of drugs were developed a long time ago and have been in use for many years. These are called the first-generation sulphonylureas. Others, termed second-generation, have been developed more recently and generally have greater potency, although they are not necessarily more effective in achieving better glycaemic control. The rate of absorption and hence activity of some of the sulphonylureas is delayed by the presence of food and this has implications for when the tablets have to be taken. Most need to be taken half an hour before meals so that absorption is not delayed and the beta cells can be stimulated to deal with the intake of food. Some of the drugs within the group are eliminated (i.e. excreted) by the kidneys, either unchanged or else as metabolized products which remain active. Some, on the other hand, are changed or metabolized into inactive compounds by the liver, before being eliminated. People with DIABETIC NEPHROPATHY or any other from of kidney impairment cannot be treated with sulphonylureas which are excreted in an active form. Many clinicians prefer to avoid using these drugs altogether in these circumstances and recommend insulin treatment instead. This may also be the case for elderly people, who are more likely to have altered renal function, particularly a high renal threshold for glucose, and who are also considered to be at greater risk of severe, sulphonylurea-induced hypoglycaemia.

Types of sulphonylureas, their properties and daily dosages

	Half life (hours)	Duration of activity (hours)	Daily dosage (mg)	Tablet size (mg)	Number of doses per day	Active compounds excreted by kidneys	Inactive compounds secreted by kidneys	Comments
FIRST GENERATION SULPHONYLUREAS								
Chlorpropamide	24–28	24–27	100–500	100 or 250	1	Yes	No	Now regarded as obsolete
Tolbutamide (Rastinon®, Glyconon®, Pramidex®)	4–8	6–12	500–3000	500	2–3	No	No	–
Tolazamide (Tolanese®)	4–7	12–24	100–1000	100 or 250	1–2	Yes	No	–

SECOND GENERATION SULPHONYLUREAS

Glipizide (Glibenese®, Minodiab®)	1–5	up to 24	2.5–20	2.5 or 5	1–2	No	No	–
Gliclazide (Diamicron®)	6–15	up to 24	40–320	80	1–2	No	No	–
Glibenclamide (Daonil®, Euglucon®)	10–16	up to 24	5–20	2.5 or 5	1–2	Yes	Yes	–
Glimepiride (Amaryl®)	5–8	about 24	1–6	1, 2, 3 or 4	1	Yes	Yes	–
Gliquidone (Glurenorm®)	12–24	up to 24	15–120	30	2–3	Yes	Yes	–

It is thought that the effect of sulphonylureas on insulin secretion operates within a fairly narrow range and the maximum benefit for an individual may occur at a lower level than the dose recommended by the drug manufacturer. Hence, at the start of treatment, the lowest possible dose is usually prescribed. A number of other drugs may interact with sulphonylureas, including some 'over-the-counter' remedies such as aspirin, intensifying their effect. The main risk from this is that of HYPOGLYCAEMIA. Drugs that have been implicated include:

- alcohol: less likely with modest intake but alcohol can have other side-effects (*see* below)
- aspirin and other salicylates: familiar painkillers and blood-thinning drugs
- azapropazone (Rheumox®): a non-steroidal anti-inflammatory drug (NSAID) used for rheumatoid arthritis, severe gout, ankylosing spondylitis
- cimetidine (Algitec®, Dyspamet®, Galenamet®, Tegamet®, Zita®): used for digestive disorders, e.g. acid reflux, acid
- chloramphenicol: antibiotic used in various preparations to combat bacterial infections
- clofibrate (Atromid-S®): used to treat hyperlipidaemia (raised blood levels of lipids or fats)
- co-trimoxazole: combined antibiotic preparation used in the treatment of urinary tract infections
- cyclophosphamide (Endoxana®): used in chemotherapy to treat some malignant conditions
- fluconazole (Diflucan®): antifungal agent used to treat fungal infections
- miconazole: antibacterial and antifungal agent used in various preparations to treat infections

- monoamine oxidase inhibitors: various drugs used in special circumstances to treat severe depression, anxiety or phobia
- phenylbutazone (Butacote®): an NSAID used only in hospital to treat severe arthritis and other serious inflammatory conditions
- probenecid (Benemid®): used to treat gout and sometimes combined with antibiotic therapy
- ranitidine (Zantac®): used to treat ulcers in the stomach and gut
- rifampicin (Rifadin®, Rifater®, Rifinah®, Rimactane®, Rrimactazid®): antibiotic used to treat serious bacterial infections, especially tuberculosis and, in other preparations, as a protection against meningitis
- sulphinpyrazone (Anturan®): used to treat gout
- sulphonamides: prevent bacterial growth and used to control infections
- tetracyclines: a large group of antibiotics used to treat infections
- trimethropim: antibacterial agent used in various preparations to treat infections
- warfarin and other drugs containing coumarin: blood-thinning agents used to prevent and treat heart and circulatory disorders.

Any drugs already being taken by a person newly diagnosed with diabetes will influence the type of treatment which is suitable. Likewise, antidiabetic medication being taken will need to be considered before any medications are prescribed for other conditions. Anyone who is worried about possible drug interactions should seek medical advice, especially before buying and using 'over-the-counter' remedies.

Apart from HYPOGLYCAEMIA, side-effects associated with sulphonylureas are generally rare and mild. However, one well-known disadvantage is that they tend to cause weight gain and increased hunger and there may be more than one cause for this. Increased insulin secretion itself may encourage weight gain as the hormone is anabolic, that is, it promotes the building up of body tissues. With improved control of blood glucose levels, less glucose is excreted and more is available to be stored as fat. Sulphonylureas are highly effective in banishing unpleasant diabetic symptoms that may have been endured for a considerable time. The person feels better and it may be that he or she has a renewed appetite and eats more. It has also been suggested that some people may overeat in the mistaken belief that in this way they can avoid hypoglycaemia. Most people with Type 2 diabetes (for whom sulphonylureas are designed) are already overweight or obese at the time of diagnosis. Hence this group of drugs is most appropriate for the minority who are either underweight or of normal weight, in whom weight gain would be less of a problem and in whom there are no other contraindications ruling out their use.

Other, generally mild, side-effects include slight stomach/ digestive upset at the start of treatment, skin rashes and headaches. These symptoms may improve with time. Some sulphonylureas (especially chlorpropamide), may cause a flushing of the face when alcohol is drunk. If any side-effects are experienced, they should be reported to the diabetes clinical team or doctor and if necessary a change of drug may be suggested.

Meglitinides: Repaglinide (Novonorm®)

Repaglinide (Novonorm®) is the first of a relatively new group of non-sulphonylureas which has a fast-acting effect upon insulin secretion. Its metabolic action is somewhat different to that of the sulphonylureas but it has been shown to be highly effective in lowering blood glucose levels. Repaglinide is designed for use only when a meal is about to be eaten and it is ideally taken 30 minutes before eating. It has a short half-life of less than 60 minutes and acts very rapidly to lower blood glucose levels after a meal has been consumed. Evidence suggests that there may be a lower risk of severe HYPOGLYCAEMIA with repaglinide compared to sulphonylureas. Studies also suggest that only a modest weight gain is associated with the use of this drug. Repaglinide is metabolized by the liver and most is excreted in *bile*, hence there is minimal involvement of the kidneys. However, it is not normally recommended for people with significant liver or kidney disease. Repaglinide is designed to be used as monotherapy or in combination with metformin, if there is still insufficient control of blood glucose levels. It provides an alternative to sulphonylureas for people with Type 2 diabetes for whom dietary and lifestyle measures are insufficient. However, it allows for greater flexibility since it is only taken when a meal is to be eaten. Repaglinide is only suitable for people who retain sufficient beta cells able to produce insulin. Since its use is associated with some weight gain, it is probably most suitable for those of normal weight.

There are a number of drugs that interact with repaglinide:

- ACE inhibitors: a group of drugs used to treat heart conditions and high blood pressure
- alcohol
- anabolic steroids: hormonal type drugs used to promote the build up of body tissues and to treat certain forms of anaemia

- azole antifungal drugs used to treat fungal infections
- beta-blockers: drugs used to treat heart conditions, anxiety, hypertension, and migraine
- contraceptive pills
- corticosteroids: hormonal preparations used to treat disorders of the adrenal glands and inflammatory conditions such as rheumatoid arthritis
- danazol (Danol®): used to treat heavy periods, endometriosis and some breast disorders
- erythromycin: antibiotics used to treat many bacterial infections
- monoamine oxidase inhibitors (MAOIs)
- non-steroidal anti-inflammatory drugs (NSAIDs): used for inflammatory conditions such as rheumatoid arthritis
- octreotide (Sandostatin®): used in hospital to treat pituitary gland and pancreatic tumours
- phenytoin (Epanutin®): used in hospital to treat irregular heartbeat and epileptic seizures
- rifampicin
- sympathomimetics: drugs used to treat respiratory disorders such as bronchitis and asthma and also in emergencies for shock and acute low blood pressure
- thiazide diuretics: used to treat some heart conditions and high blood pressure
- thyroid hormones: used to treat disorders of the thyroid gland.

Apart from HYPOGLYCAEMIA, side-effects associated with the use of repaglinide are generally slight and are similar to those which may occur with sulphonylureas, with possible visual disturbances also having been reported. Anyone experiencing side-effects should report these to their

diabetes clinical care team. Repaglinide tablets are available in 0.5 mg, 1 mg and 2 mg dosages and it is usual to
start with the smallest dose, increasing this to a maximum
4 mg single dose (i.e. 2×2 mg tablets), if necessary. The
maximum daily dose is 16 mg (i.e. 2×2 mg tablets, 4 times
a day, taken before meals). People who are transferring
from another form of antidiabetic medication are usually
started on an initial 1 mg dose of repaglinide.

Biguanides: Metformin (Glucophage®)

The only drug in this group licensed for use in the UK is
metformin (chemically known as dimethylbiguanide). The
drug has a complex metabolic activity and works in a
number of different ways, but it does not increase insulin
secretion. Its principal effect is to inhibit gluconeogenesis and so reduce the manufacture of glucose by the liver.
In addition, it promotes the action of insulin so that more
glucose is taken up from the circulation into muscles and
tissues and its effects appear to be mainly within cells,
beyond the receptor sites. Evidence suggests that metformin
also lowers blood lipid levels (triglycerides and cholesterol)
but this effect is variable. The combined effects of
metformin are anti-hyperglycaemic, and it improves glycaemic control in people with Type 2 diabetes. The drug
is not associated with weight gain, and in fact there is a
tendency for weight loss to occur, especially during the
early course of treatment. Hence it is often recommended
for those who are overweight, unless there are existing
conditions which rule out its use.

Metformin has a half-life of two to three hours and it is
absorbed into the blood from the small intestine. It is not
metabolized by the liver but is excreted unchanged by the

kidneys. This means that it is not suitable for those with any kidney impairment such as DIABETIC NEPHROPATHY, and people receiving metformin require occasional monitoring of their renal function. This involves checking for the presence of protein in the urine or raised creatine levels in the blood. (Creatine is a metabolic product normally excreted in urine.)

The main serious risk from treatment with metformin is the occurrence of an acute metabolic complication known as LACTIC ACIDOSIS (*see* Chapter 7), but this is very rare. Lactic acid is produced from glucose, most commonly by skeletal muscle but also in the brain, red blood cells and kidneys when oxygen is absent, in order to supply energy for vital functions. Lactic acid is composed of lactate and hydrogen ions, and usually lactate is extracted by the liver, heart and kidneys. However, in conditions of severe oxygen shortage, there can be an excessive build-up of lactic acid, resulting in lactic acidosis. This most commonly occurs when the tissues are starved of oxygen (tissue hypoxia) as a result of, for example, life-threatening shock or cardiac failure. However, it can also occur (very rarely) in diabetes and as a complication of metformin treatment because of the way the drug works metabolically. It is, however, considered to be a very small risk. It only occurs if the drug should happen to be used in the presence of some unsuspected underlying condition, especially kidney impairment. (The kidneys excrete metformin and impairment may lead to a build-up of the drug and hence an increased risk of lactic acidosis.) For this reason, people with any impairment of the kidneys, liver or heart or who might be at risk of tissue hypoxia, or who abuse alcohol, are not suitable for treatment with metformin. Those who are prescribed the drug are carefully monitored, especially for any development of impaired organ function.

A common side effect with metformin is gastrointestinal upset which can include nausea, vomiting, diarrhoea, wind and appetite loss. To avoid or minimize these problems, the tablets should either be taken with meals or immediately after eating. Quite often, the problem resolves as the person becomes accustomed to the drug but occasionally, symptoms persist or are unpleasant enough to necessitate a change of treatment. There may be a slight, metallic aftertaste in the mouth, and absorption of vitamin B_{12} and folate (B_9) can also be affected, but not severely enough to cause problems. It is, however, sensible to eat plenty of foods containing these vitamins, if receiving metformin treatment and advice on this will be given by the clinical dietitian. Tablets are supplied in 500 mg and 850 mg dosages and the usual starting dose is 500 mg twice each day. The maximum dose is one 850 mg tablet twice daily or one 500 mg tablet three times a day. Tablets should always be taken at meal times. Metformin may also be combined with other oral antidiabetic drugs or, less commonly, with insulin therapy. Excretion of metformin is affected by cimetidine (a drug used to treat ulcers, acid stomach and pancreatitis) and a lower dose or a different medication is needed in people who are receiving this drug.

Alpha-glucosidase Inhibitors (Acarbose)

Acarbose (Glucobay®) is the only drug in this group licensed for use in the UK but others are likely to become available in the future. Acarbose works in the small intestine by inhibiting alpha-glucosidases, which are enzymes that break down carbohydrates into glucose. Hence there is less glucose available to be absorbed into the blood and peaking of blood sugar levels is reduced. Acarbose is designed to be used immediately before or at the start of a carbohydrate-containing meal. The drug is metabolized by bacteria within the gut into inactive products which are eliminated in faeces or absorbed into the blood and eventually excreted by the kidneys in urine. Acarbose may be used as monotherapy before any other drugs are tried or it may be combined with other antidiabetic agents. Used alone, it does not cause HYPOGLYCAEMIA but it may add to the hypoglycaemic potential of sulphonylureas or insulin, if used in combination.

Gastrointestinal upset is a common side-effect with acarbose and its manifestations include wind, diarrhoea and bloating. These symptoms occur because more carbohydrate passes unchanged into the large bowel where it is subjected to fermentation by gut bacteria. Symptoms are experienced by about one-third of those taking acarbose, especially by people being treated with higher dose regimes. However, symptoms tend to subside with time as the person adjusts to the drug. Strict avoidance of sugar in the diet and very minimal dose increases, introduced gradually, help to minimize unpleasant gastrointestinal symptoms. However, if symptoms persist, it may be necessary to try alternative medication. Acarbose does not cause weight gain and so is highly suitable for people with Type 2 diabetes, who are likely to be overweight. However, it can cause a rise in the plasma blood levels of certain liver enzymes and so it is not suitable for people with any impairment of liver function. Due to its gastrointestinal effects, it is also ruled out for people with various bowel disorders, including ulcerative colitis, inflammatory bowel disease, and obstructions of the bowel, such as hernias, irritable bowel syndrome and so on. It is not prescribed for people with severe kidney disorders or impairment of renal function.

The tablets are supplied in 50 mg and 100 mg dose sizes. The starting dose is 1×50 mg tablet taken with the first mouthful of the main daily meal. After two weeks, if the drug is well tolerated, the dose is increased to introduce a second 50 mg tablet with a different meal. This is followed for a further two weeks and then a third 50 mg tablet is introduced, taken with the remaining meal. If there are adverse side-effects, the dosage is dropped back to the previous level. After six weeks, the dose may be further increased in a gradual way, possibly introducing the 100 mg tablet with one meal. The maximum permitted dose is 3×100 mg tablets, each taken separately with one main meal. Acarbose may interact with the following drugs:

- pancreatic enzymes: used for disorders of the pancreas when there is a lack of digestive enzymes
- cholestyramine (Questran®): used for relief of diarrhoea in biliary disorders and to treat hyperlipidaemia (raised blood fat levels)
- neomycin: an antibiotic used to treat infections within the intestine.

Surgical Forms of Treatment for Diabetes: Pancreatic and Islet Cell Transplants

Transplantation of either the whole or part of the pancreas is occasionally performed, most often in the USA. It is generally carried out in people with Type 1 diabetes who have advanced DIABETIC NEPHROPATHY and require a kidney transplant. In these circumstances, a double transplant of a kidney and pancreas may be performed. As with all such operations, a major factor is the need to use powerful immunosuppressive drugs to prevent the organs from being rejected. These drugs cause side-effects and also increase the risks of cancer and diabetes itself.

Immunosuppression carries with it a greatly increased risk of serious infections, especially cytomegalovirus. The reasoning behind combined operations is that since the patient requires immunosuppression for the kidney transplant, it may be worthwhile to attempt to transplant a pancreas at the same time, if the organ is available. Although this is high-risk surgery, most centres do not carry out pancreatic transplants alone but prefer to attempt the double operation as a means of saving life. About one-third of transplants fail within the first year and up to half fail after five years. However, if successful, transplantation can result in a higher quality of life, removing the need for insulin treatment and abolishing the risk of severe HYPOGLYCAEMIA. However, a return to completely normal metabolic control is usually not achieved.

Transplants of islet cells have not so far proved possible for many complex reasons, including the need for immunosuppression. However, it is hoped that a breakthrough will occur, enabling cell transplants to become a reality and this is a field in which there is a considerable amount of ongoing research.

4

INSULIN TREATMENT

Insulin treatment is essential for people with Type 1 diabetes. They have insulin-dependent diabetes mellitus (IDDM), the former, descriptive name for this form of the syndrome. They require what is, in effect, insulin replacement therapy because by the time they are diagnosed, they are producing no insulin of their own. In these circumstances, insulin treatment is both life-saving and necessary throughout life. As we have seen, people with Type 2 syndrome (non-insulin dependent diabetes mellitus, NIDDM) may manage successfully with other forms of treatment but a significant proportion eventually require insulin. Often, this is simply a reflection of the progressive nature of Type 2 syndrome, in which effective insulin activity within the body tends to decline to a low level. In other cases, glycaemic control with antidiabetic drugs may have been poor for some reason, or there may be complications present such as liver or kidney disease which necessitate the use of insulin. Sometimes, people with Type 2 diabetes are managed with a combination of tablets and insulin. It is important to realize that a partial or complete change to insulin does not mean that Type 2 diabetes is getting worse or that the person has somehow 'failed' with other treatments. Most of those who change to insulin feel a great deal better, find it much easier to cope with than they expected, and are happy to continue with the treatment. Insulin therapy can only be successful if the person receiving it feels secure and confident about every aspect of their treatment. There is always plenty of time allowed for discussion and explanation at the diabetes clinic so that all concerns (such as 'needle phobia') can be addressed. Support and encouragement are considered to be very important and part of the ongoing work of the diabetes clinical care team. Before discussing insulin treatment in more detail, it is useful to look more closely at the nature of the insulin itself.

The Nature of Insulin

There are four main types, or species, of insulin, according to the (mammalian) source from which each is obtained.

- Beef or bovine insulin is obtained from the pancreas of cattle and is one of the earliest forms of insulin to be used in human treatment. Its structure differs from that of human insulin in three amino acids (proteins) and it is now more or less obsolete. It is still produced for people who have used this type of insulin for many years and for whom change is unsuitable, for one reason or another. However, it is no longer prescribed for people newly diagnosed with diabetes.
- Pork or porcine insulin is derived from the pancreas of pigs and it differs from human insulin in only one amino acid in its structure. Semi-synthetic porcine insulin, which is chemically modified in the laboratory, is also available. Porcine insulin continues to be used by a minority of people with diabetes.
- Human insulin is produced in the laboratory by genetic engineering:
  - from a proinsulin (a precursor insulin molecule);

- ○ from a proinsulin precursor made by genetically modified yeast organisms (labelled 'pyr' on insulin bottles);
- ○ from some other method of genetic engineering (labelled 'ge' on insulin preparations).

Hence no human insulin used in treatment is in any way taken from human bodies, either living or dead.

- Human insulin analogues are copies of the human insulin molecule and are substances not found in nature but ones that have been recently developed by genetic engineering. There are two types:

  - ○ insulin lispro, in which the position of two amino acids (lysine and proline) have been changed (lys + pro = lispro);
  - ○ insulin asparte, in which aspartic acid has been substituted for the amino acid, proline, at position B28 on the insulin molecule.

In the past, animal insulin preparations, particularly those derived from beef, incorporated a number of impurities and people who were treated with them usually produced insulin antibodies as an immune response. Occasionally this caused localized reactions, particularly around injection sites. Modern, purified animal insulins are not associated with these reactions, which are now very rare. Since beef insulin differs from human insulin in three amino acids, a relatively higher dose is generally required in treatment. People being changed from beef to human insulin, are usually given an initial dose which is 20 per cent lower than the one they were receiving before. This is to lessen the risk of HYPOGLYCAEMIA. Switching from pork to human insulin is generally more straightforward but may also require dose adjustment.

When manufactured human insulins were first developed and started to be used more widely, some problems were experienced by a minority of people switching from animal insulins. These mainly related to HYPOGLYCAEMIC UNAWARENESS in that some people reported a lessening in intensity of the early warning signs of a hypoglycaemic episode. Other problems included depression, sleeplessness, irritability, forgetfulness and lethargy, which were reported by a small number of people. It should be stressed that the majority of people had, and continue to have, no problems with human insulins and the issue remains a controversial one. It is vital that the person being treated feels confident about the species of insulin being used and, after full discussion, the choice rests with the individual concerned.

Types of Insulin, according to Duration of Action

Insulin is classified according to its duration of action, with some preparations designed to be quick-acting while others exert their effects over a longer period of time. In general, among the rapid-acting types, human insulin is the fastest species to take effect, followed by porcine and then bovine. Insulin is delivered by means of a subcutaneous injection (i.e. beneath the skin) and in order to begin to work, it must be absorbed into the circulation. The location of the injection site slightly influences the rate at which this occurs and absorption is most rapid from the abdominal area (i.e. around the middle). Massaging the injection site, exercise and heat also promote absorption and smaller quantities of insulin are taken up more rapidly than larger amounts. These are factors other than the design of the insulin itself that exert some effect upon speed of action.

Very Quick-acting Insulin Analogues (Lispro and Asparte)

These are newly developed, clear insulins which are the most rapidly absorbed of all the types that are available and the quickest to reach a peak of activity (effect). They begin to act 10 to 20 minutes after being injected and reach a peak of activity in one hour. The duration of their effect is three to four hours. Insulin analogues provide an alternative to the more familiar, QUICK-ACTING CLEAR INSULINS and can be used just before, or even immediately following a meal. Early evidence suggests that they may reduce the risk of severe, NOCTURNAL HYPOGLYCAEMIA in some people and improve overall glycaemic control. However, they are not suitable for everyone, and in some circumstances their rapid action can be a disadvantage and so they are always used cautiously. A well-known type of lispro insulin is called Humalog®.

Quick-acting Soluble or Clear Insulin

This is the traditional type of rapid-acting insulin of which there are several different formulations. Their number include Hypurin® Bovine Neutral, Hypurin® Porcine Neutral, Pork Velosulin®, Humulin® S, Human Velosulin® and Human Actrapid®. These begin to work in about 30 minutes and reach a peak of activity in one to three hours. Their duration of action is about four to eight hours, and soluble insulins should ideally be injected half an hour before a meal is to be eaten. They are mainly used to regulate the meal-time glucose intake and are generally superimposed upon 'background' injections of longer-lasting types of insulin. (Sometimes the two are given together as a pre-mixed preparation: *see* INSULIN MIXTURES below.)

Intermediate-acting Cloudy Insulins
These take a longer time before they begin to work and have a more prolonged period of activity. There are two types.

Isophane Insulins
These are among the most widely used types and preparations include Hypurin® Bovine Isophane, Hypurin® Porcine Isophane, Pork Insulatard®, Humulin® 1 and Human Insulatard®. They begin to take effect after about two hours, with a peak of activity lasting between four and twelve hours. The maximum duration of their effect is between 22 and 24 hours, and isophanes are used to provide 'background' or basal insulin, usually in combination with quick-acting preparations.

Lente Insulins
These have similar properties and examples include Hypurin® Bovine Lente, Humulin® Lente and Human Monotard®. These begin to exert an effect after about two hours with a peak of activity lasting for between six and fourteen hours. Like isophanes, the total duration of effects is around 22 to 24 hours and they are usually used in combination with fast-acting preparations.

Long-acting Cloudy Insulins
These are the longest-lasting insulin preparations and examples include Hypurin® Bovine Protamine Zinc, Hypurin® Bovine Lente, Humulin® Zn and Human

Ultratard®. These are more variable than other insulins with a peak of activity ranging between eight and twelve hours and total effects that may last up to 28 hours.

Insulin Mixtures

These are pre-mixed preparations, usually of quick (clear) and intermediate (cloudy) insulins. Most mixtures consist of a combination of clear and cloudy isophane insulins but, less commonly, lente insulin may be used as the longer-acting component. The ratios of the two insulins vary:

Clear: Cloudy Ratio	Examples
10:90	Human Mixtard® 10; Humulin® M1
20:80	Human Mixtard® 20
30:70	Human Mixtard® 30; Pork Mixtard® 30; Hypurin® Porcine and Biphasic Isophane® 30:70 mix
40:60	Human Mixtard® 40
50:60	Human Mixtard® 50; Humulin® M5

In the UK, the most commonly used mixture is the 30:70 one.

Injecting Insulin

Everyone who needs insulin is shown how to inject it during their first visit to the diabetes clinic. Plenty of time is allowed to discuss all the available options and to choose a delivery method with which the person feels comfortable and confident. Time is also allocated for demonstration and practice of the technique. Fear of needles is a problem that is well recognized by clinical care staff and not something which is treated lightly or laughed at but regarded as a difficulty that must be worked through and overcome. This is always achievable. A minority of people have a true needle phobia and this may take a little more time to deal with. A probable approach would be to suggest that the person undertakes a programme of behavioural therapy, which is normally successful in overcoming phobias. It is never the case that someone is forced into accepting insulin treatment without the necessary help to make this possible, or left to get on with it on his or her own. Full support is given from the start and continues to be available.

Although the idea of self-administered injections may seem daunting at first, for most people this rapidly becomes a matter of routine which is dealt with as easily as, for example, brushing one's teeth. An easily available site, such as the thigh or abdomen, will probably be suggested for the first injection and advice will be given on how often to change the site in order to avoid soreness or possible slight tissue damage. Hands should be washed prior to giving the injection and the person is usually advised to take a good pinch of skin and insert the needle at an angle of 90 degrees to its full depth. The plunger is then gently and firmly depressed to expel all the insulin. After five seconds, the needle is then carefully withdrawn.

Insulin Delivery Devices
Insulin given to treat diabetes has to be delivered by means of a subcutaneous injection, that is, one beneath the skin,

and the most usual sites are the thighs, upper arms, abdomen or buttocks. (Insulin used for diagnostic or emergency treatment, for example to test insulin sensitivity, is a special type which is only administered in a clinical setting and is injected or infused intravenously, i.e. via a vein.) The needles used to deliver insulin are very short and extremely fine and when correctly given, injections are not painful. There are three main ways in which insulin is given.

- Conventional method by means of a needle and syringe. Insulin is drawn up into the syringe by inserting the needle into the vial or bottle through a stopper. Vials may contain a single type of insulin or mixtures. Disposable plastic syringes, especially for insulin, are available in various sizes. (*See* DRAWING UP INSULIN below.)
- A pen device and cartridge which contains the insulin. Cartridges may contain 1.5 ml or 3 ml of insulin and are changed when empty. Disposable needles are used with pen devices.
- A pre-loaded pen with integral needle, all of which is disposed of once empty.

There are various pen devices available, some of which are designed to be used with particular ranges of insulin and each may have slightly different operating instructions. The manufacturer's instructions must always be read carefully. Some more sophisticated pens (e.g. Diapen® 1 and 2) have an automatic injection mechanism and a device for regulating the depth to which the needle is inserted. Usually, these more sophisticated pens are also the most expensive! The most popular pens are called Novopen® and BD® pen. Syringes, insulin pens and cartridges are available free on prescription, but at the present time, needles have to be paid for, although this is something which is being challenged.

Drawing up Insulin (Vials and Syringes)

Drawing up the correct dose of insulin is another task which may seem worrying at first but once again, plenty of time is set aside for the demonstration and practice of this so that the person can feel confident about being able to do it accurately. It may take time to gain the necessary confidence and so the process is made easier by breaking it down into stages and clearly demonstrating each stage. Written, step-by-step instructions for use at home are provided by diabetes care staff and so there is no need for the person to commit it all to memory straight away. Before starting, always check that your insulin preparations are the correct ones prescribed for you and that they are within their use-by date. Instructions are made as easy to follow as possible and are usually similar to the following.

For a Single Dose of Insulin

1. Wash hands thoroughly.
2. Roll the bottle of insulin between your hands or gently tip it from side to side to make sure that the contents are evenly mixed, but do not shake the bottle.
3. Take the syringe, with needle attached, and holding it upside down, pull up the plunger to the line on the syringe corresponding with the insulin dose. This allows a volume of air equal to the amount of insulin to enter the syringe.
4. Pick up the insulin bottle with one hand, keeping it upright. With the other hand, insert the needle attached to the syringe through the rubber stopper of the bottle. Push

down the plunger of the syringe so that the air previously drawn up enters the bottle. (This makes the next stage easier to perform.)

5. With the needle and syringe in place, turn everything upside down so that the point of the needle is now surrounded by fluid insulin. Draw back the plunger to the level slightly beyond (i.e. more than) the required insulin dose to take up the insulin.

6. Gently tap or flick the side of the syringe so that any air bubbles present rise to the top. Depress the plunger slightly to expel the air bubbles, stopping at the level of the exact insulin dose.

7. Double-check that the dose is correct and withdraw the needle from the stopper of the bottle. The insulin dose is now ready to use.

Drawing Up and Mixing Clear and Cloudy Insulin

1. Wash hands thoroughly.

2. Gently mix each bottle of insulin to be used, as in Step 2 above. Do not shake the bottles.

3. Take the syringe with the needle attached and holding it upside down, draw up a volume of air equal to the dose of CLOUDY insulin as described in Step 3 above.

4. Take the bottle of CLOUDY insulin and hold it upright. Insert the needle through the rubber stopper and inject the air just drawn up into the CLOUDY insulin bottle. Withdraw the needle.

5. Holding the syringe upside down, pull back the plunger to draw up a volume of air equal to the CLEAR insulin dose.

6. Take the bottle of CLEAR insulin and keeping it upright, insert the needle through the rubber stopper.

Inject the air just drawn up into the CLEAR insulin bottle.

7. Turn everything upside down and make sure that the needle point is surrounded by the CLEAR insulin. Pull the plunger back to a level slightly beyond (i.e. more than) the required insulin dose.

8. Gently tap or flick the syringe to make any air bubbles rise to the top. Depress the plunger slightly to the level of the exact CLEAR insulin dose.

9. Double-check that the dose is correct and withdraw the needle from the CLEAR insulin bottle. Keep the syringe inverted with the needle point uppermost.

10. Take the bottle of CLOUDY insulin and turn it upside down. Insert the needle of the syringe through the rubber stopper of the CLOUDY insulin bottle.

11. Ensure that the needle point is surrounded by CLOUDY insulin and draw back the plunger to the exact dose required, to take up the CLOUDY insulin. (If too much is taken up by accident, withdraw the needle from the bottle, expel all the contents of the syringe down the sink and start again! Do not try to inject the extra back into the CLOUDY insulin bottle as the two insulins will already have become mixed within the syringe. The CLOUDY insulin bottle will become contaminated with CLEAR insulin if you try to do this.)

12. Withdraw the needle from the CLOUDY insulin bottle. The mixed dose of CLEAR and CLOUDY insulin is now ready for use.

People who are new to insulin treatment and who choose the syringe and vial method, are usually taught how to draw up a single dose of one type of insulin at first. Mixing insulins in the manner described above is usually introduced a little later once the person feels completely confident about the procedure.

Insulin Treatment Regimes

People being treated with insulin are asked to inject their insulin at certain times of the day, in order to regulate their levels of blood glucose. To a certain extent, the timing of the injections is an attempt to mirror the pattern of insulin secretion that occurs in normal health. As noted previously, insulin is normally secreted at a low level throughout the day, with sharp increases in response to the intake of food. This insulin is released into the portal blood system (the circulatory network that serves the abdominal digestive tract or lower gut, spleen, pancreas, gall bladder and liver). Levels of insulin reaching the systemic circulation (blood system supplying other tissues and areas of the body) are normally about half that of those in the portal circulation. Injected insulin is delivered into the systemic circulation so that levels are high here and initially lower in the portal system, which is the opposite to the situation that exists in normal health. At first sight, there are several other disadvantages in the crude system of injecting insulin, compared to the exquisitely finely-tuned response that occurs in normality! These include:

- difficulties in matching the insulin dose to actual glucose levels and especially in controlling fasting plasma glucose levels. Once given, the insulin dose cannot be reduced or retrieved. Snacks are often needed to prevent HYPOGLYCAEMIA.

- relative inflexibility of a system relying on injections to cope with day-to-day changes in food intake, levels of exercise and other variables
- normal, day-to-day variability in rate of absorption of insulin doses and imprecise action and duration of effects of manufactured insulin
- other individual factors, such as medical conditions, illnesses, stress, etc., which can influence the absorption, action and effects of injected insulin.

In fact, one expert in diabetes, speaking about the deficiencies of insulin therapy compared to normal health, has said that 'insulin is injected in the wrong place, at the wrong time and in the wrong amounts' (Gale, 1996). In spite of this and for all its perceived deficiencies, he goes on to state that, remarkably, insulin therapy achieves good glycaemic control in the majority of those who receive it and most people respond extremely well!

It is recommended that injections of clear or fast-acting insulins are given half an hour before meal times and this is also the case for cloudy insulins used during the day. Cloudy or long-acting insulins used before going to bed to last through the night do not need to be taken before eating. Quick-acting lispro and asparte insulins can be taken between 15 and 5 minutes before a meal.

There are several different types of insulin treatment regime.

Once-daily Insulin

This regime is only used in elderly or infirm people, where the aim is to prevent HYPOGLYCAEMIA. Good control of blood glucose cannot be achieved with only one injection of insulin. The types of insulin used are either an intermediate cloudy lente preparation such as Human Monotard® or a long-acting type like Humulin® Zn. The type of person for whom this regime might be recommended is someone elderly who has Type 2 diabetes.

Twice-daily Insulin

Free-mixed or pre-mixed preparations may be used, combining short-acting, clear insulins or fast-acting insulin analogues with intermediate-acting isophane or lente cloudy insulins. This is the most popular and commonly used regime, with the injections usually given before breakfast and before the evening meal. However, there are limitations, and snacks may need to be eaten between meals and before going to bed to avoid HYPOGLYCAEMIA. This is because of the way the short and longer-acting insulins work and the timing of the peaks of their activity, which may enable some 'gaps' in optimal cover to occur. Free mixing of the insulins, which is usually recommended for people with Type 1 diabetes on this regime, allows for greater flexibility in insulin cover as doses can then be adjusted. Pre-mixed combinations are more likely to be suitable for those with Type 2 diabetes.

Multiple Daily Injections and the Basal Bolus Regime

These consist of three doses of short-acting, clear insulin (or three of rapid-acting such as lispro), injected half an hour before each main meal, combined with one injection of intermediate-acting cloudy insulin (isophane or lente), given at about 10 p.m. to last through the night and into the following day. The pattern is intended to reflect that which occurs in normal health, and these regimes may be used to treat both types of diabetes, but are particularly suitable for those with Type 1 syndrome. If a pen device is used, as is commonly the case, it is known as the Basal Bolus regime. Multiple injections, coupled with frequent checking of blood glucose levels (*see* Chapter 5, HOME BLOOD GLUCOSE MONITORING), form the basis of 'tight' control of glycaemia. An advantage of this regime is that it can be adapted to allow for greater flexibility in the timing of meals, and eating occasional larger or smaller meals can be accommodated, both by means of ADJUSTING INSULIN DOSES.

One practical disadvantage, apart from having to self-administer four injections each day, is the possible need to test the effect of each dose by monitoring blood glucose levels. Blood glucose tests may be carried out on rising in the morning (to check the effect of the cloudy insulin given the previous night), and then two hours after each meal to monitor the clear insulin doses. In practice, once a person has settled into the Basal Bolus regime and if he or she has a regular, daily routine (in terms of size of meals and their timing), it may be possible to reduce the number of blood glucose tests. By carrying out fewer tests but at different times on consecutive days, it is possible to obtain a reasonably good picture of what is happening to blood glucose levels. However, frequent testing is usually necessary when the desired aim is to achieve tight control of glycaemia. The main drawback with multiple injection regimes and one which is, understandably, a cause of anxiety, is that there is an increased incidence of HYPOGLYCAEMIA.

Continuous Subcutaneous Insulin Infusion (CSSI)
This is a specialized system, not in common use, which is offered by a few larger diabetes centres which are able to

provide 24-hour back-up care. Fine tubing connects a pump to a needle inserted beneath the skin of the abdominal wall. The battery-powered pump is programmed to deliver constant, clear insulin at a basal level with pulses of the hormone at meal times. One of the main problems is blockage of the tubing and also, there can be soreness at the site of implantation. The needle can easily become dislodged because the device is worn continuously and serious problems such as DIABETIC KETOACIDOSIS can arise quite quickly if there is an interruption in the insulin supply.

Combined Insulin and Drug Therapy

Combining oral, antidiabetic drugs with insulin is an appropriate treatment for some people with Type 2 diabetes. Sometimes, this type of regime is transitory and the person may eventually transfer to insulin alone. In other cases, combination therapy may be continued for some considerable time. Two types of antidiabetic drug (sulphonylureas and metformin) are most commonly combined with insulin.

Sulphonylureas and Insulin

Usually, sulphonylureas are taken during the day and cloudy insulin (isophane) is injected at night or in the morning. The results of some studies suggest that half the normal insulin dose is sufficient with this combination, at least in the initial stages of treatment.

Metformin and Insulin

Once again, metformin is taken during the day and cloudy (isophane) insulin is injected at night and/or in the morning. Studies suggest that there is a lower risk of weight gain with this regime compared to insulin therapy alone, in Type 2 diabetes. It may also provide better control of blood glucose levels than twice-daily insulin alone. It is thought to be a particularly suitable therapy for overweight people with Type 2 syndrome, in whom further weight gain is obviously undesirable.

Selecting the Insulin Regime and Starting Doses

Choosing an insulin regime depends upon a number of different factors which include the type of diabetes, the clinical needs and the preferences of the person concerned, taking into account the daily routine and lifestyle and whether tight control is the desired aim. It is important to realize that both the regime and the insulin doses may change over time from that which is suggested at the start of treatment. Insulin regimes and doses work best when they are adapted to individual needs, depending upon the results of blood glucose monitoring, and so they may require modification with the passage of time. Most people are started on insulin on an out-patient basis at the diabetes clinic and this includes the minority who have been newly diagnosed with Type 1 syndrome. The exceptions are those who are ill at the time of diagnosis (usually people with Type 1 diabetes), who present with pronounced symptoms, marked hyperglycaemia and moderate to severe ketonuria. Anyone whose condition gives cause for concern is normally admitted to hospital and given the appropriate treatment, which may include intravenous infusion with insulin. Once the diabetes has been controlled and the person feels better, he or she is normally referred to the diabetes clinic (generally within the same hospital), so that a suitable insulin regime can be started before returning home.

There are no hard-and-fast rules about the starting dose of insulin, which varies according to individual need. However, most clinics try to keep starting doses small to minimize the risk of HYPOGLYCAEMIA. The usual procedure is to help the person to self-administer the first insulin dose during the course of the initial clinical appointment, allowing plenty of time for demonstration and practice. A starting, daily adult dose would usually lie in the range of 16 to 24 units of insulin, divided between two injections. On the first day, having self-administered the first injection at the clinic, the person is sent home with instructions on the time to give the evening and following morning doses. Recognizing that giving these first home injections can seem daunting, most clinics provide clear, illustrated written instructions and a helpline that can connect the person with someone who can give support and advice, should the need arise. Often, the first insulin doses are pre-mixed or single insulins to make matters easier in these early stages. The person is also likely to have received advice about suitable meals and quantities of food to be eaten. He or she may have been shown HOME BLOOD GLUCOSE MONITORING and HOME URINE TESTING. Usually, a follow-up appointment is made for the next day or within a few days, so that progress can be fully discussed and help provided with any difficulties.

Obtaining and Storing Insulin

People with diabetes who are being treated with oral medication and/or insulin, are entitled to free prescriptions for all the drugs that they may need. This not only includes their diabetes medication but prescriptions for other types of drugs as well. As mentioned previously, insulin delivery devices are also included in this although needles have to be bought. However, some clinics make their own arrangements about the supply of needles and in any case, the cost is relatively small. The situation with regard to needles may change in the future.

Most people receive their first insulin supplies, testing strips etc. (for blood glucose/urine monitoring) from their diabetes clinic, which may be based at the nearest hospital or local health centre. The quantities supplied may vary between clinics. A communication will be made to the person's family doctor giving details of the type of insulin and other supplies that the patient requires. Repeat prescriptions can then be obtained from the doctor's surgery. It is recommended that spare insulin supplies should be stored in the vegetable compartment or door of the refrigerator. The insulin that is in current use should be kept at room temperature but not left in direct sunlight or in a hot place such as a shelf above a heater. A cartridge or vial of insulin should always be examined before use and a quick check made to ensure that it is of the correct type and dose and within the manufacturer's expiry date. It is helpful to know the type and name of your insulin and to have this recorded on a personal diabetes card (supplied by the clinic) which is kept readily to hand for reference. If insulin looks peculiar in any way, for example discoloured or with the wrong consistency, it should be discarded and not used.

Disposal of 'Sharps'

Some diabetes clinics operate a disposal scheme for used insulin equipment and all give advice on how to deal with this. A device is available, free of charge, which clips off the needles and stores them and is able to hold about two years' supply. Syringes, vials, cartridges and pens can be placed in an empty household container, such as a margarine tub, and the lid taped down when full. The container can either be taken to the clinic or surgery for special disposal, or, if no local service is available, put out with household rubbish.

Adjusting Insulin Doses

In order to achieve a better and more flexible control of diabetes treated with insulin, it is necessary to adjust the doses from time to time. There are various reasons why this adjustment may be required.

• The starting insulin regime may be inadequate and results of blood tests may indicate that better control could be achieved by increasing or decreasing the overall dose.
• The person's lifestyle and/or work commitments, e.g. working shifts or regular international travel across time zones, may make it essential to adjust insulin doses.
• Regular or irregular adjustment may be needed to accommodate planned or unplanned EXERCISE and activities, hot weather (at home or on holiday), stressful periods, times of illness (e.g. colds, flu, stomach bugs), religious festivals and fasts and other special occasions (*see* Chapter 11).

It is very useful if the affected person can learn to adjust his or her insulin doses as this gives greater individual control of the diabetes. However, it is well recognized that many people find this difficult and prefer to leave decisions about their insulin dose to the diabetes care team. Diabetes staff are happy to undertake this and no one needs to feel under pressure to alter doses on their own if they are not confident about doing this. However, it is considered to be important to educate people about self-adjustment as part of the general process of learning about diabetes. The first step is for the person to understand the mode of operation of the insulins he or she is using (i.e. short- or long-acting or both) and how and when they may overlap in their effects. Studies suggest that among insulin users, there is, in fact, a great deal of misunderstanding about even the basic facts. Also, among those who do undertake self-adjustment, there are two extremes of people – those who alter doses too frequently without a clear need to do so and those who do not alter them enough!

Although there are no definitive rules, there are some general guidelines that are usually followed when adjusting insulin doses.

- Regular HOME BLOOD GLUCOSE MONITORING (HGBM) must be carried out and accurate readings of blood glucose levels recorded at different times of the day. In this way a picture of the effects of each insulin dose is obtained and can be analysed and understood.
- A pattern of regular, adverse readings (i.e. lying outside the target range) should have been obtained before altering an insulin dose. The exception is if adjustment is being done in advance as a planned measure, for example to accommodate strenuous exercise.
- Alterations in dose(s) should be small.
- Only one dose at a time should be altered and the effects monitored over a few days by means of HBGM. (People using pre-mixed preparations of two insulins should seek advice.)
- Cloudy insulin should be altered infrequently, i.e. no more than every two or three days.

It must be appreciated that a reading of a blood glucose level relates to the effects of the previous insulin dose, not the one that is coming up. If an adverse blood glucose reading has been obtained regularly over a period of days, then the relevant insulin dose cannot be altered until it once more becomes due, which is usually on the following day. One of the most common mistakes that is made is to alter the next insulin dose that is due on the same day, in the mistaken belief that this will correct the problem, when in fact, this only makes matters worse! It is especially important that those on a multiple injection, Basal Bolus regime appreciate the need to adjust the relevant insulin dose as it is all too easy for the whole scheme of control to go awry.

- Never withhold an insulin dose that is due, even in the event of a low blood glucose reading or a hypoglycaemic attack. The 'hypo' should be treated (*see* Chapter 6) to restore blood glucose levels and the due dose given as usual. This is because the episode has been caused by previous events and cannot be helped by withholding the next insulin dose.
- If in doubt about altering any insulin dose, seek expert advice.

Side-effects of Insulin Treatment (other than Hypoglycaemia)

The most common side-effect of insulin treatment is weight gain, which is thought to arise due to three possible causes. Firstly, insulin is known to have an anabolic (body-building) effect. In the second place, when good glycaemic control starts to be achieved due to insulin therapy, less glucose is lost in urine. This glucose is potentially available for storage as fat and it is possible that this accounts for some weight gain. Thirdly, insulin treatment makes people feel better and they usually find that it rapidly banishes unpleasant symptoms. A renewed sense of health and wellbeing may simply mean that the person recovers his or her appetite and feels able to eat more than before. In a minority of people, especially in those with Type 1 syndrome who have lost weight prior to diagnosis, regaining weight is a desirable outcome. However, for those who are already overweight, especially those with Type 2 diabetes, further weight gain is obviously unwelcome. Usually, if it happens at all, the gain occurs quite soon after insulin treatment has been started and then ceases. Careful attention to diet at the beginning of treatment, along with increasing levels of exercise, may prevent or minimize weight gain. However, it may be advisable for those with Type 2 diabetes to follow a weight loss diet from the start.

Other, rare, side-effects occasionally occur, including water retention affecting the feet and lower legs, deterioration in existing RETINOPATHY (eye disease), and neuritis (painful inflammation of nerves). The first two are usually short-lived and subside and improve with time, but neuritis can be persistent and require more prolonged treatment of the symptoms.

Intensive Insulin Therapy in People with Type 1 Diabetes

Intensive insulin therapy, or 'tight' control, based upon a multiple injection/Basal Bolus regime, attempts to maintain blood glucose at near normal levels for most of the time. Research studies have shown that good control of glycaemia, achieved through intensive insulin treatment, reduces the risk of MICROVASCULAR COMPLICATIONS of diabetes, namely, RETINOPATHY, NEUROPATHY and NEPHROPATHY. Also, when these complications are present, insulin therapy may in some cases slow their rate of progression. Unfortunately, these desirable outcomes are counter-balanced by a serious disadvantage, which is an increased incidence of severe episodes of HYPOGLYCAEMIA, that is, attacks which require the intervention and assistance of other people. Further disadvantages are the need for a high degree of motivation on the part of the person concerned, in order to carry out frequent monitoring of blood glucose levels and to self-administer several injections each day.

From a clinical point of view, there are certain groups of people for whom intensive treatment with insulin is inadvisable. They include those who already experience episodes of severe HYPOGLYCAEMIA and people who are unable to recognize or who do not experience the early-warning signs of an attack. It is also unsuitable for people with major or advanced tissue damage resulting from diabetic complications and those with heart disease or other serious conditions. Finally, intensive insulin therapy is unsuitable for children under the age of 13 because repeated episodes of hypoglycaemia can harm the developing brain.

Tight Control of Glycaemia in People with Type 2 Diabetes

Tight glycaemic control in Type 2 diabetes may be achieved using SULPHONYLUREAS and/or insulin. Studies suggest that rigorous treatment for those with this syndrome results in a similar reduction in the risks posed by MICROVASCULAR COMPLICATIONS. Once again, the major disadvantage is an increased incidence of severe HYPOGLYCAEMIA, as well as weight gain.

5

MONITORING GLUCOSE LEVELS

Home Blood Glucose Monitoring (HBGM)

The ability to monitor blood glucose levels at home is vital for those with Type 1 diabetes and may well be essential for people with Type 2 syndrome as well, especially if they are being treated with SULPHONYLUREAS or insulin. One of the main advantages of HBGM is that it enables people to be in better control of their diabetes, when combined with adjustment of insulin doses. HBGM enables HYPOGLYCAEMIA to be detected. This is very reassuring for many people, especially for those at risk of more severe 'hypos', that is, those whose diabetes is being tightly controlled.

How to Carry Out an HBGM Test

General guidance for performing HBGM is listed below, although the instructions given by your own diabetes clinic should be followed.

1. Wash hands with warm water and soap and dry thoroughly.
2. Select lancet and/or finger-pricking device and extract a test strip from its container.
3. Prick the side of a finger tip (avoiding the thumb and index finger) and massage gently to obtain a good drop of blood.
4. Place the strip over the drop of blood and move it sideways to cover it completely with blood. Make sure that

you accurately follow the instructions for using the strip with a meter.

5. Cover the puncture with a small piece of clean gauze or cotton wool hold in place for a few minutes.
6. 'Read' the blood glucose using the chart or meter and note the result in the diary provided by your clinic.
7. Take some glucose if the reading is at or below 4 mmol/l, but follow specific guidance on this given by your clinical care team.
8. Whatever the result, do not miss out your next dose of insulin or sulphonylureas.

HBGM Procedure: Potential Difficulties

Although HBGM is desirable, there are several well-recognized potential difficulties connected with the procedure.

• A finger-prick blood sample must be obtained for each test and people may find this uncomfortable and unpleasant, especially because it has to be carried out on a regular daily basis. Someone newly receiving insulin treatment may be asked to perform four tests a day but usually, the number can be reduced once a pattern of readings has emerged.

• Blood glucose levels are assessed by using enzyme-impregnated strips or sticks which are available free on prescription. These can either be 'read' visually by matching the colour on the strip to a chart, or else with the aid of a specially designed meter. There are more than 12 types of meter available, some with large print displays or an audio output for people with sight or hearing difficulties. However, meters are not available on prescription and must be bought by the patient. Costs vary considerably, depending upon the sophistication of the meter and the facilities it provides, such as memory and the ability to link with a computer. People sometimes think that they need to buy an expensive, elaborate meter, when in fact a much more simple device would equally suit their needs. Clinical staff are always happy to advise about meters and have first-hand experience of the different types that are available. Some clinics make their own arrangements and can provide meters free of charge, at least to some of their clients. The people most likely to benefit would be those newly diagnosed with Type 1 diabetes. Meters vary in their operational instructions, which must always be followed meticulously. Each meter will use a particular type of test strip. Although training in the use of meters is given at diabetes clinics, some people find the equipment difficult to use when on their own at home.

- Specially designed, very fine blades or needles known as lancets are available free on prescription for HBGM. Like insulin needles, after they have been used, these must be placed in a container with a lid and disposed of safely, in accordance with local arrangements and advice given by the diabetes clinic. Hand-held devices are available which can be pre-loaded with a lancet. When held against the side of a finger and triggered, the point of the lancet shoots into the surface of the skin making a pin-prick and making it easier to obtain a drop of blood. These devices are not available on general prescription, although some clinics may make their own arrangements and be able to provide them for some of their patients. Whatever the method used, many people find finger-pricking the most difficult part of carrying out HBGM and some find it so unpleasant that they do not test for blood glucose as often as they should.

- Obtaining accurate results from HBGM depends upon attentiveness at all stages of the procedure, from obtaining a 'clean' drop of blood to correct use and storage of test strips, meters and charts. Once obtained, each reading must also be noted in a 'monitoring diary' provided by the clinic. It is known that errors can easily be introduced at any stage, with potentially serious consequences if the end result is an inappropriate alteration of an insulin dose.

- Some people, understandably, feel that HBGM is one task too many on top of the daily necessity of having to self-inject insulin. It is not uncommon for there to be major discrepancies between the results presented by the patient and those (based on glycated haemoglobin, *see* CLINICAL MONITORING OF BLOOD GLUCOSE LEVELS below) obtained by the clinic. As noted above, people may test too infrequently and then, as a clinical appointment approaches, be tempted to invent good results! The only way around this is if the patient can learn to appreciate the benefit to his or her own health of regular HBGM.

- People suffering from physical or intellectual impairment, mental illness or depression, and young children may need extra help and encouragement with HBGM. It is likely that family and/or carers will need to be involved, as they probably are already with insulin injections. Carers and families can feel a considerable burden of responsibility in performing these tasks, which also impinge upon their own freedom, tying them to the routine of the person with diabetes. All this requires understanding, help and support and a good relationship with diabetes clinical staff so that problems can be discussed openly. In the same way, the physically disabled person with diabetes may feel frustrated about not being able to manage HBGM and insulin injections and may struggle with his or her dependency.

The Glucose Oxidase Reaction

The HBGM test is based on a biochemical reaction brought about by an enzyme called glucose oxidase. The test strips are impregnated with this enzyme and a reduced dye. When a drop of blood is placed on the strip, the glucose it contains is oxidized by the enzyme (i.e. oxygen is added), to produce gluconic acid and hydrogen peroxide. The amount of hydrogen peroxide produced is directly related to the amount of glucose present in the blood. The hydrogen peroxide reacts with the dye in the strip to produce a colour which is dependent upon the amount of glucose that was present in the drop of blood.

Interpreting the Results: What is an Acceptable Range for Blood Glucose Levels?

Once again, diabetes clinical care staff will assess what is a reasonable range of blood glucose levels for each person and it is their guidance that should be followed. Ideally, good control of blood glucose is the desired aim which means levels lying between 4 and 7 mmol/l between meals (and 9 mmol/l after a meal). Diabetes UK uses the phrase 'make four the floor' meaning that the level should not fall below 4 mmol/l as there is then a risk of HYPOGLYCAEMIA. In practice, it is difficult to keep within the ideal range all of the time, for a number of different reasons, sometimes because of complex metabolic causes over which the individual has little control. Hence it is important to understand that a result outside the range does not represent an individual failure or fault and should not be a matter of guilt about something the person thinks he has or has not done. What is important is for the person to know what action needs to be taken if a consistent pattern of high or low readings has emerged, by, for example, eating a snack or altering an insulin dose as required, or taking avoiding action if a single result indicates a risk of hypoglycaemia.

Clinical Monitoring of Blood Glucose Levels: Testing for HBA1c

Some of the blood samples taken on clinical visits are subjected to a different sort of laboratory testing which measures the amount of glycated haemoglobin or HBA1c. HBA1c is produced by the glycation of haemoglobin. The biochemical process of glycation is the attachment of glucose molecules to the amino part of proteins. Haemoglobin is the important respiratory substance in red blood cells which contains a pigment that is responsible for the red colour of blood but which also carries oxygen around the body. Glycation occurs in other tissues as well, causing damage and alteration of protein structures. It is part of the process known as cross-linking of proteins which leads to the production and accumulation of substances known as Advanced Glycation End products or AGEs. The process of glycation occurs without the activity of enzymes and is proportionate to the mean, average concentration of glucose in the blood. Since the amount of glycated haemoglobin in the blood, in relation to normal haemoglobin, is proportional to the average glucose levels that have existed in previous weeks, it provides a useful assessment of glycaemia in diabetes. It is known that in normal health, the proportion of HBA1c is between 4 and 6 per cent. A measurement of HBA1c in diabetes is made at least twice a year on routine clinical visits. Along with the person's own record from HBGM, it allows a good assessment of overall glycaemic control to be made, and together the results provide the basis for clinical staff to suggest changes to an insulin or drug regime, if required. HBA1c can be considered to be complementary to the daily recording of HBGM. The results need to be interpreted carefully by experts since there are some circumstances in which 'false' readings can be obtained, for example in some conditions that affect the red blood cells themselves.

It is worth noting that glycation and cross-linking of proteins with the accumulation of AGEs are favoured by hyperglycaemia, particularly when this goes undetected and persists for a long time, as is often the case in Type 2 diabetes. It is believed that this process contributes to the tissue damage seen in some of the LONG-TERM COMPLICATIONS of diabetes, such as changes to the walls of blood vessels in arterial and heart disease. Restoration of good control of glycaemia, especially early on in the course of diabetes, helps to slow down glycation and cross-linking and thus prevent protein and tissue damage. However, the process is also associated with ageing and the tissue changes that occur as people get older, whether diabetes is present or not.

New Developments in Blood Glucose Monitoring

New ways of measuring blood glucose levels, with the aim of making the process easier to perform for people with diabetes, are continually being researched and developed. There have been many projects on the development of new sophisticated meters which can give a reading for blood glucose in a matter of seconds and have other facilities as well. New non-invasive devices that do not require a blood sample are also being attempted. Some of these use laser or infra-red technology but they still need to be calibrated quite frequently and this requires a blood sample. However, one new device, worn like a wristwatch and being developed in the USA, measures glucose levels in the interstitial fluid (a clear fluid present between cells and tissues) without piercing the skin. At the present time, these new devices are expensive and not widely available but it is expected that they will eventually be introduced. A non-invasive method of measuring blood glucose would make the whole process of HBGM much more acceptable, and so more likely to be performed. This in turn would help people to manage their diabetes more effectively.

Home Urine Testing (HUT)

Testing a urine sample for the presence or level of glucose is a far more crude method of assessing glycaemic control. It has the advantage of being simple to perform and is non-invasive and so there is no discomfort involved. This makes it a more acceptable test than HBGM and hence one which is more likely to be carried out. Unfortunately, there are several disadvantages. The presence of glucose in urine is dependent upon the person's renal threshold. As mentioned previously, this is the level or concentration above which glucose ceases to be 'recycled' by the kidneys back into the bloodstream so that it passes into the urine. The normal level at which this occurs in adults is 10 mmol/l but it varies a great deal, not only between individuals but at different stages in one person's life. Children tend to have a low renal threshold and may have glycosuria (sugar in the urine) in the absence of diabetes. Elderly people are far more likely to have a high renal threshold. Glycosuria may be absent in the presence of hyperglycaemia and elevated HBA1c. The concentration of the urine and the quantity of fluid that has been drunk can affect the HUT reading, and, particularly important, a urine test cannot detect HYPOGLYCAEMIA. In spite of its limitations, HUT can provide useful information and reassurance, especially for people with Type 2 diabetes. It is inadequate as a testing method for tightly controlled diabetes or where there is a risk of hypoglycaemia.

How to Carry Out a Urine Test
In order to test for sugar in the urine, special strips are used which are coated with a reagent that changes colour according to the amount of glucose present. Testing is simply a matter of collecting a urine sample and dipping the strip into it or alternatively, holding the strip in the urine stream. The test is timed and the colour compared with colours on a chart, indicating the amount of sugar present. Urine test strips are available free on prescription and there are various types, including some which are specially designed for people who are colour-blind. The timing and frequency of testing will depend upon individual advice given by diabetes clinical staff. Results of the tests should be noted in a diary or on a chart so that a record is kept which can be analysed when necessary.

Testing Urine for Ketones
Although this test is carried out in a similar way to that described above, that is, by dipping a specially prepared stick or strip into a urine sample and noting a colour change, the

reasons for testing are quite different. In this case, it is not glucose that is being looked for but ketones to detect ketonuria. Ketonuria is a feature of Type 1 diabetes and is a warning sign of the risk of DIABETIC KETOACIDOSIS (DKA). People with newly diagnosed Type 1 diabetes often test positive for ketones in their urine, but these usually disappear quickly with the initiation of insulin treatment. In fact, ketonuria usually improves even before hyperglycaemia. Hence testing urine for ketones may well be suggested for people in this position and carrying it out provides early positive proof of the efficacy of insulin therapy. The other main circumstance in which the test is useful is during periods of occasional illness (*see* Chapter 11, COPING WITH ILLNESS AND INFECTION). Urine testing for ketones is carried out using test strips or sticks (called ketosticks) which can detect acetoacetate. A colour change occurs which is then compared with colours on a chart supplied by the diabetes clinic. The colour indicates whether there are no ketones, a minute amount, or small, medium or large quantities present. The person will receive advice on whether action needs to be taken and what form this should take: if the results indicate a potential risk, hospital admission may be necessary to stabilize the diabetes.

6

HYPOGLYCAEMIA

Many people think that hypoglycaemia is a feature of diabetes, but it is in fact a side-effect of certain forms of treatment for the condition, notably insulin and sulphonylurea therapy. Hypoglycaemia is more common in people with Type 1 diabetes, 10 per cent of whom experience at least one serious episode each year, requiring hospital treatment, in addition to less severe attacks. The good news is that these episodes are almost always successfully treated and the person is usually quickly restored to normal health. In spite of this hypoglycaemia is, quite understandably, the most feared side-effect of insulin treatment. Unfortunately, as we have seen, the incidence of severe 'hypos' increases with tight glycaemic control in Type 1 diabetes. This is the main limiting factor in intensive insulin therapy and achieving good glycaemic control. Intensive treatment is highly desirable since it reduces the risks of diabetic complications, but the fear of hypoglycaemia makes many people with diabetes hesitate about intensive therapy.

People with Type 2 diabetes who are being treated with SULPHONYLUREAS and/or insulin may also experience hypoglycaemia, but for most the attacks are less frequent and not so severe. However, very severe episodes of hypoglycaemia are a rare but recognized hazard of sulphonylurea treatment, especially in elderly people. These attacks may prove fatal in extremely unusual circumstances. When this has occurred, it has usually been connected with one of the longer-acting sulphonylureas, although any one of this group of drugs has the potential to cause hypoglycaemia. This risk means that longer-acting sulphonylureas are not normally prescribed for elderly people. It is thought that the action of sulphonylureas in suppressing glucose production by the liver is the main reason why these drugs may cause hypoglycaemia. Elderly people appear to be particularly susceptible to this effect. Other high-risk situations which may exacerbate the hypoglycaemic potential of sulphonylureas, are interactions with other drugs, including alcohol, and metabolic stresses caused by periods of infection or illness (*see* Chapter 11).

The Definition of Hypoglycaemia

Hypoglycaemia is said to exist if the level of glucose in the blood falls below 3.3 mmol/l. However, Diabetes UK has recommended that 4 mmol/l should be the recognized basal level below which there is a risk or likelihood of hypoglycaemia. This has become the 'working level' adopted by diabetes clinics and upon which their advice to patients is based.

Immediate Causes of Hypoglycaemia

In the short-term, hypoglycaemia has two main causes relating either to the supply of carbohydrate or to the amount of available insulin. Very often, a hypo is caused either by inadequate carbohydrate intake as in a missed, late or small meal, or by an increase in the rate at which glucose is utilized due to a greater demand for energy. The latter situation generally results from increased physical exercise or activity, which can be something as simple as gardening or spring-cleaning. Alternatively, a hypo may be caused by excess treatment. This may either be the direct result of too much insulin being injected or, in the case of SULPHONYLUREAS, an excess dose provoking a greater than normal release of insulin from beta cells. In both cases, the net effect can be a fall in the circulating level of glucose, and if this descends too low, the development of hypoglycaemia. Other immediate causes or factors which can contribute to an attack include a higher than normal intake of alcohol, change of injection site, and hot weather (which affects insulin/glucose metabolism). It may be that there is no obvious cause for a particular 'hypo' but after recovery, it is always worthwhile to undertake a mental review of previous events and to try and discover the reason why it may have happened. Usually, some seemingly minor factor, possibly something that has not been a problem before, turns out to be the most likely cause. The purpose of the 'postmortem' is to try and avoid a recurrence in the future, even though this may not always be easy.

Longer-term Causes of (Recurrent) Hypoglycaemia

There are a number of other, longer-term causes of hypoglycaemia, which generally cause it to be recurrent, rather than a single episode that happens due to one recent event. These include:

- the 'honeymoon period' in Type 1 diabetes, when there may be an initial apparent recovery of islet cells (invariably short-lived) following the initiation of insulin treatment. The honeymoon period usually comes to an abrupt end, often coinciding with a period of illness. A person in this position is usually carefully monitored and maintained on a minimal dose of insulin in order to avoid hypoglycaemia, rather than insulin treatment being stopped altogether.

- alteration or change in insulin sensitivity, for example, the resolution of INSULIN RESISTANCE following childbirth or after withdrawal of steroid therapy
- development of kidney or severe liver disease, underactive pituitary or thyroid gland, Addison's disease, disorders affecting absorption of nutrients, e.g. coeliac disease
- severe weight loss or eating disorders.

These disorders may affect different people in various ways with regard to hypoglycaemia. Treatment of the primary cause, rather than hypoglycaemia as such, usually removes or lessens the risk of attacks.

Events within the Body during Hypoglycaemia

As blood glucose levels fall during hypoglycaemia, the body responds by activating a sequence of counter-regulatory hormones to try and reverse the decline. The hormones are secreted in a particular sequence, namely, glucagon (from pancreatic alpha cells), adrenaline and noradrenaline (secreted by an area of the adrenal glands called the medulla whose normal function is to prepare the body for 'fright', 'flight' or 'fight'), cortisol (released by the cortex of the adrenal glands and involved in glucose metabolism and stress responses), and growth hormone (from the pituitary gland). Glucagon, adrenaline and noradrenaline stimulate the processes of glycogenolysis and gluconeogenesis (*see* Chapter 1, THE BACKGROUND TO DIABETES) which results in the production and release of glucose from the liver. Cortisol and growth hormone are less involved in acute hypoglycaemia but are important in the later restoration of glucose levels. However, when secretion of these hormones is impaired for any reason, as in pituitary gland disorders (this gland controls adrenal production of cortisol) and Addison's disease, which affects the adrenal glands themselves, hypoglycaemia is likely to occur. Addison's disease can itself be a complicating feature of Type 1 diabetes.

When insulin or SULPHONYLUREAS are needed to treat diabetes, the counter-regulatory hormonal responses are often inadequate to prevent hypoglycaemia.

Clinical Grades of Hypoglycaemia and Symptoms

In clinical, medical terms, four grades of hypoglycaemia are recognized.

Grade 1: its existence can be detected biochemically but it does not produce symptoms.

Grade 2: produces only mild symptoms and can be easily treated by the affected person.

Grade 3: produces more severe symptoms and requires the assistance of another person.

Grade 4: very severe, producing unconsciousness, coma and/or convulsions and requiring emergency treatment in hospital.

In practice, people who experience hypoglycaemia or who are considered to be at risk are given advice on how to treat three categories designated mild, moderate and severe. The treatment for these is described below.

The symptoms of hypoglycaemia can be attributed to two main causes. Involvement of the autonomic nervous system (the part of the nervous system that is not under conscious control) and the release of hormones from the adrenal glands, produces 'fright', 'flight' and 'fight' symptoms. These typically include anxiety, trembling, sweating, shivering, pallor, palpitations and a raised heartbeat rate, and dizziness. These are called adrenergic symptoms. The brain is very soon affected by the inadequate energy supply, as blood glucose levels fall during hypoglycaemia, producing the second category of neuroglycopenic symptoms. These include inability to concentrate, confusion, irrational, aggressive or uncharacteristic behaviour, speech disturbance, refusal to co-operate, drowsiness, and eventual loss of consciousness. If treatment is not provided, there is a risk of convulsions and eventual permanent brain damage or, in extreme circumstances, death. A third group of symptoms, which do not directly belong to either category but are commonly experienced, include hunger, disturbance of vision, transient headache, and feelings of weakness.

In experimental conditions of induced hypoglycaemia, adrenergic symptoms are produced first at a higher level of blood glucose while neuroglycopenic ones begin as the level continues to descend. Many people learn to recognize adrenergic symptoms as an early warning of hypoglycaemia and are able to take action to rectify the situation. However, there are circumstances (*see* below) where this is not the case, and in any particular hypoglycaemic episode not all symptoms may be present, or there may be neuroglycopenic ones appearing at the same time as adrenergic ones, so that the situation is not always clear cut.

Advice and Treatment for Hypoglycaemia

Family and friends, as well as the affected person, need to learn how to recognize hypoglycaemia and what action to take and this forms an important part of education about diabetes. A person subject to 'hypos' should always carry some form of readily absorbed sugar with them such as glucose tablets, sugar lumps, soft sweets, honey, chocolate or a sweet drink. Action at an early stage quickly restores the person to normal and averts the development of further symptoms.

Mild Hypoglycaemia

Symptoms most commonly experienced are the adrenergic ones or those in the non-specific category. Treatment is simply a matter of taking in a small amount (10 g) of rapidly absorbed glucose, such as four glucose tablets or sweets, two teaspoons of honey, or a small sweet drink. An affected person should sit down quietly for five minutes and when feeling better should eat a snack containing carbohydrate (e.g. a sandwich or fruit), or have the next meal, if it is due. This is to prevent a recurrence of the hypoglycaemia. It may be advisable to check the blood glucose level after eating to ensure that this is returning to a safe level, and the next insulin dose should be given as normal. If symptoms arise while driving (or operating machinery), find a safe place to pull in and stop the car. Remove the keys from the ignition and move to the passenger seat. Do not start driving again until fully recovered.

Moderate Hypoglycaemia

Brain function is affected and typical symptoms include confusion, irritability and odd or aggressive behaviour, sometimes mistaken for drunkenness. The affected person requires help from someone else but may try to refuse aid. The most effective treatment, as long as the person is conscious, is to persuade him or her to take some sugar in liquid form. A thick glucose gel is available from diabetes clinics and this can be squirted into the mouth. Alternatively, honey, treacle, a sweet drink or sugar dissolved in warm water are equally good alternatives. They should be spooned into the person's mouth, and even if he or she is resisting swallowing, some will be absorbed through the membrane lining the mouth and this will improve symptoms. Once this occurs, the person usually becomes more co-operative and will then accept some more. When he or she feels better, a carbohydrate-containing snack or meal should be eaten, as for mild hypoglycaemia. It is advisable to monitor blood glucose levels for a time, following recovery.

Severe Hypoglycaemia (in Type 1 Diabetes and Insulin-Treated Type 2 Diabetes)

This stage is marked by unconsciousness and obviously, the person requires outside aid in order to recover. The standard treatment is an injection of glucagon beneath the skin, this being the hormone that stimulates the release of glucose by the liver (*see* Chapter 1, THE BACKGROUND TO DIABETES). The glucagon is supplied in an easy-to-use kit, containing simple and clear instructions and is available from diabetes clinics. Usually, a family member is shown how to use the kit as part of the general education about diabetes offered by the clinic, but anyone can administer the injection in an emergency. Once the person regains consciousness, he or she must be given a small amount of readily absorbed glucose by mouth, followed by a carbohydrate-containing snack or meal, once he or she has recovered sufficiently to be able to eat. Blood glucose levels should be monitored during the recovery period and the person may feel the need to rest for the remaining part of the day.

If the glucagon injection does not work (and it may take up to 15 minutes to have an effect) and the person dremains unconscious, or there is any other cause for concern, emergency medical help should be summoned.

Severe, Sulphonylurea-induced Hypoglycaemia (in Type 2 Diabetes)
This is a medical emergency requiring expert treatment in hospital. In sulphonylurea-treated patients, recurrence of the hypoglycaemia after initial recovery is common and so the person has to be closely monitored. The mainstay of treatment is dextrose given by intravenous infusion and this may be required for several days. Glucagon is not an appropriate treatment for sulphonylurea-induced hypoglycaemia because one of its effects is to stimulate the release of insulin, which is likely to make the situation worse. Although rare, this type of hypoglycaemia is serious and especially worrying if it occurs in older people.

Nocturnal Hypoglycaemia
Hypoglycaemia occurring during sleep is quite common in Type 1 diabetes and often produces no symptoms. It is particularly worrying for parents when it occurs in young children who can be at risk of impairment of brain function if the attacks are frequent. For this reason, parents are given special and detailed advice on how to reduce the risks and the appropriate action to take. In adults, nocturnal hypoglycaemia sometimes produces symptoms of night sweats or the person may have a headache on waking. It is advisable to carry out HOME BLOOD GLUCOSE MONITORING between 2 and 3 a.m. for a few nights (in accordance with clinical advice), if it is suspected that nocturnal hypoglycaemia is occurring. It is

usually necessary to alter the dose of evening insulin and recent research suggests that it is the dose of short-acting clear insulin that is the most critical in nocturnal hypoglycaemia. Also, it is often necessary to eat a carbohydrate-containing snack before going to bed. It is very important to be extremely careful about alcohol consumption, especially if nocturnal hypoglycaemia is a problem. Even a modest amount of alcohol (which would not normally be considered excessive) can cause problems in susceptible people and alcohol-related hypoglycaemia can be triggered many hours after the drinks have been consumed.

It is thought that unrecognized, recurrent nocturnal hypoglycaemia may make a significant contribution to the problem of HYPOGLYCAEMIC UNAWARENESS (see below). Also, hypoglycaemia may be more likely to develop at night because normal physiological responses to falling blood glucose levels are reduced during certain (slow-wave) stages of sleep.

Factors that Affect Hypoglycaemia

There are various factors, closely connected with the necessary treatment of diabetes with insulin, which can affect hypoglycaemia.

Effect of Recurrent Hypoglycaemia and Hypoglycaemic Unawareness

Both insulin therapy for more than five years and lifelong diabetes itself, are likely eventually to cause defective counter-regulatory hormonal responses to hypoglycaemia, especially those involving glucagon. Normal brain function is critically dependent upon a good supply of glucose from the circulation at all times. The glucose is transported to the brain by specialized transporter proteins called GLUT 1. It has been found that previous and recurrent hypoglycaemia (such as nocturnal hypoglycaemia) alters the rate at which this occurs during subsequent attacks. There is an increased rate of glucose transfer to the brain during subsequent episodes of hypoglycaemia, which is an adaptive response. The effect of both defective hormonal responses and adaptive changes in glucose transfer to the brain can be a loss or decreased awareness of hypoglycaemic symptoms. This is known as hypoglycaemic unawareness. When this is present, a person becomes aware of symptoms only at lower blood glucose levels or he or she may not notice them at all. Hence there is far less time to take restorative action and a much greater risk of loss of consciousness and the development of a severe attack. This is the situation that arises more frequently in tightly controlled, intensively treated Type 1 diabetes. Quite often, awareness of warning symptoms can be restored by returning to a less intensive treatment regime in which blood glucose is maintained at a higher level.

Effect of Insulin Type and Species

In the UK, there has been a considerable amount of debate about whether particular types of insulin may cause hypoglycaemic unawareness. This arose because a few people reported a decreased awareness when they changed from animal to human insulin. Although there is no scientific evidence for any problem with human insulin in this respect, it is known that individuals can react differently to particular type of insulin and that changes in dose may be needed if there is a switch from one kind to another. Diabetes clinical staff are always ready to listen to people's concerns about insulin and are happy to supply a particular type or suggest a change if this would seem to be beneficial.

Prevention of Hypoglycaemia

During the course of a lifetime's treatment with insulin (or SULPHONYLUREAS), it is difficult entirely to prevent the occasional episode of hypoglycaemia. However, there are measures that can be taken to minimize the risk. Some of these have already been mentioned previously but they can be summarized as follows.

- Take insulin doses at the times recommended by your diabetes clinical care team.
- Eat meals and snacks on time, again according to clinical advice.
- Monitor blood glucose levels regularly to check the effects of each insulin dose and to ensure that injections match food intake.
- Always carry a supply of glucose with you.
- Be aware of the possible effect of changing the injection site on the rate of insulin absorption – advice on this is given at the diabetes clinic.
- Always have a snack or meal before driving. On longer journeys, check your blood glucose before and during the travel period. Make regular stops for food and rest. If you experience warning signs of a hypo, stop the car in a safe place, switch off the engine, remove the keys from the ignition and move to the passenger seat to take your glucose.
- Carry diabetes identification with you at all times so that your condition will be recognized, should you have a hypo.

- Inform family, friends, work colleagues, and so on, about the possibility of hypoglycaemia. Explain what they need to do to help, should it prove necessary.
- Be aware of the effects of EXERCISE, adjust insulin dose and/or eat a carbohydrate containing snack before starting, in accordance with clinical advice. If the exercise is unplanned, eat some extra carbohydrate.
- Take extra care when travelling and crossing time zones (*see* Chapter 11).

7

ACUTE METABOLIC COMPLICATIONS OF DIABETES

A number of well-recognized complications are associated with diabetes and these can be grouped into two main categories. The first category of acute metabolic complications, although relatively uncommon, consists of life-threatening medical emergencies requiring immediate admittance to hospital for intensive treatment. They may sometimes prove fatal. There are two conditions in this category: diabetic ketoacidosis (DKA) and hyperosmolar syndrome (HONK). The second category of well-recognized complications that are associated with diabetes consists of LONG-TERM COMPLICATIONS and these are discussed in Chapters 8 and 9.

Diabetic Ketoacidosis (DKA)

DKA is a severe metabolic condition in which there is marked hyperglycaemia and greatly elevated levels of ketones in the blood, leading to metabolic acidosis. This means that the acidity of the blood and tissue fluids is raised to an abnormally high level due to a failure of metabolic regulation, causing serious physiological disturbance within the body. The following medical definitions of DKA have been suggested:

'Severe, uncontrolled diabetes requiring emergency treatment with insulin and intravenous fluids, with a blood ketone body concentration of greater than 5 mmol/l.' (Alberti, 1974)

* * *

'A capillary or arterial plasma bicarbonate concentration of less than 15 mmol/l.' (Krentz and Nattress, 1977)

* * *

A urinary ketostix reaction of + + or greater. (In most Accident and Emergency departments, ketones in the urine are measured using dipsticks such as ketostix. *See* Chapter 5, TESTING URINE FOR KETONES.)

DKA usually develops rapidly over a period of a few days and produces a number of symptoms and clinical signs. These include:

- excessive thirst and urination (polyuria)
- passing large quantities of urine at night (nocturia)
- rapid weight loss (due to dehydration and metabolic breakdown)
- nausea and vomiting
- muscular weakness and cramps, especially in the legs
- flushing of the face
- abdominal pain, deep
- rapid breathing (known as Kussmaul respiration, caused by acidosis)
- drowsiness and, eventually, coma.

People with DKA are quite often admitted to hospital with persistent vomiting as the most apparent symptom, in the first instance. As acidosis worsens, there is an effect upon the heart and circulation and people with severe DKA may have a rapid heartbeat, arrhythmias and hypotension (very low blood pressure) in addition to the symptoms listed above. Treatment involves skilful management in an intensive care unit and constant, careful monitoring of the person's condition. The aim is to correct the physiological imbalances accompanying dehydration, loss of electrolytes and hyperglycaemia. This involves rehydration with fluids, electrolytes and insulin, all given intravenously. As the person improves, insulin is given by subcutaneous injection and the person will be encouraged to eat normally, as soon as he or she is well enough to do so.

Unfortunately, acute and severe complications, which can sometimes prove fatal, can accompany DKA, including cerebral oedema (fluid on the brain), which is especially likely to occur in children, adult respiratory distress syndrome (ARDS), thromboembolism (thrombosis, stroke), and in rare cases increased coagulation and viscosity of the blood (known as disseminated intravascular coagulation). Also, but again rarely, an opportunistic fungal infection of the nasal passages, sinuses and brain may develop – a condition called rhinocerebral mucormycosis.

DKA is more likely to affect people with Type 1 diabetes but can, in unusual cases, occur in those with Type 2 syndrome. The overall average mortality rate in DKA is about 5 per cent of those affected, and in some cases there is an identifiable, precipitating cause. The most common precipitating factors for DKA are:

- infection (the most likely cause), underlining the importance of continuing to administer insulin doses during times of illness
- mismanagement of diabetes (connected with the above) either by the person concerned or, more rarely, by health

professionals. In most cases, the mismanagement is in not administering insulin

- previously undiagnosed diabetes (about 10 per cent of people presenting in DKA have not been diagnosed as having diabetes)
- no obvious identifiable cause.

Although DKA is a severe condition it is relatively rare and individual risks can be lessened by careful adherence to good management of diabetes.

Diabetic Hyperosmolar Non-ketotic Syndrome (HONK)

HONK has some similarities to DKA but there are also significant differences – in its development, the people affected, physiology, symptoms and rate of mortality. HONK usually develops over a period of several weeks, instead of days which is the usual case with DKA. It is characterized by very high blood glucose levels, usually greater than 50 mmol/l and often in excess of 60 mmol/l. In DKA hyperglycaemia is not so high and blood glucose levels are usually less than 40 mmol/l. In HONK there is no ketosis or acidosis, ketonuria or hyperketonaemia. Ketones are either absent from blood and urine or only present at a minimal level. This is in marked contrast to the situation in DKA. In HONK there is a high level of bicarbonate in blood plasma, usually exceeding 18 mmol/l (plasma osmolarity), whereas in DKA the level is usually below 15 mmol/l. HONK produces profound dehydration, intense thirst, polyuria, drowsiness and eventual loss of consciousness, similar signs to those of DKA. The person with HONK often responds to their intense thirst by drinking large quantities of sweet, fizzy drinks which only makes the situation worse as this contributes to hyperglycaemia and dehydration. HONK does not produce symptoms of vomiting or abnormal, Kussmaul breathing, but affected people are often admitted to hospital in an unconscious state as medical emergencies.

HONK occurs less frequently than DKA and it usually affects people with Type 2 diabetes. It is most commonly encountered in middle-aged or elderly people, and in 60 per cent of cases it occurs in those with previously undiagnosed diabetes. The mortality rate, at 30 per cent, is much higher than in DKA, and death often results from thromboembolic complications such as pulmonary embolism or stroke. As with DKA, there are a number of well-recognized pre-cipitating causes. These include infection, treatment with certain antihypertensive drugs (used to bring down high blood pressure, especially thiazide diuretics), and a high consumption of sweet drinks (understandable in those who do not know that they have diabetes).

As with DKA, a person with HONK requires specialized treatment and monitoring in hospital in an intensive care unit. The condition is managed in a similar way to DKA by reversing dehydration and loss of electrolytes and initiating insulin treatment, all by means of intravenous infusion. Once the person has recovered and is able to eat, insulin is usually given by means of subcutaneous injection. Eventually, most people who recover from HONK are able to transfer to ORAL ANTIDIABETIC DRUGS to manage their diabetes. After recovery, an attempt is made to discover the underlying cause so that a recurrence can be avoided in the future.

Lactic Acidosis

This is another rare acute complication which can arise in diabetes as a result of faulty lactate metabolism. It was particularly associated with the use of a certain type of biguanide (*see* Chapter 3, ORAL ANTIDIABETIC DRUGS) called phenformin, but has become extremely rare since this drug was withdrawn. Its occurrence now is confined to those being treated with metformin and almost all of those affected have undiagnosed kidney impairment and hence are, in fact, unsuitable for biguanide therapy.

8

LONG-TERM CHRONIC COMPLICATIONS: MICROVASCULAR DISEASES

The second category of well-recognized complications that are associated with diabetes are longer-term complications that can be divided into two sub-groups: microvascular and macrovascular diseases. These tend to develop over an extended period of time and can be severe and disabling and a cause of premature death. Good care and management of diabetes, as well as of general health, can lessen the risks.

Both Type 1 and Type 2 diabetes are associated with the development of tissue and organ complications that arise as a result of long-term insidious alteration and damage to the microvascular (small blood vessels) and macro vascular (large blood vessels) circulation. Macrovascular complications are dealt with in the next chapter.

Microvascular complications are caused by high intracellular (between cells) levels of glucose which alter certain biochemical reactions, ultimately causing changes to the walls of the small blood vessels, making them weak and 'leaky'. Structural alteration of proteins by cross-linking may also contribute to this damage (*see* Chapter 5, CLINICAL MONITORING OF BLOOD GLUCOSE LEVELS). Microvascular complications affect the eyes (RETINOPATHY and conditions arising from it), kidneys (NEPHROPATHY) and nerves (NEUROPATHY, e.g. DIABETIC FOOT DISEASE).

Retinopathy (Damage Affecting the Eyes)

Diabetic retinopathy is a degenerative condition affecting the capillaries (fine blood vessels) of the retina of the eye. (The retina is the layer that lines the back of the eye on which the 'seeing image' is formed.) Retinopathy is the most prevalent form of eye disease in diabetes and is the commonest cause of partial and complete blindness in the UK and other Western countries. Cataracts and primary glaucoma (i.e. glaucoma that develops independently) are both more likely to occur in people with diabetes. A form of secondary glaucoma can also occur as a result of advanced diabetic eye disease (a very advanced stage of retinopathy).

In essence, damage to the capillaries, which develops over a long period of time, causes these tiny blood vessels to enlarge and leak and then to proliferate. New capillaries grow in a disordered way in an attempt to compensate for, and replace, the ones that have been damaged, and this in itself causes further disruption of vision. Retinopathy occurs in both Type 1 and Type 2 diabetes but progresses differently in each form. Each type of diabetes carries a greater risk of a different stage in retinopathy than the other. However, for both types of diabetes, two factors are known to be important with regard to retinopathy. These are the length of time that the person has had diabetes and the degree of glycaemic control. Other risk factors, both for incidence and progression, are HYPERTENSION (particularly important) and, possibly, age at diagnosis of diabetes. Also significant are proteinuria (protein in urine), extent of insulin requirement and duration of treatment time. Ethnic origin may be a factor and some studies have indicated that retinopathy is more likely to occur in particular racial groups.

Good and especially 'tight' glycaemic control is known to reduce both the incidence and progression of retinopathy. However, paradoxically, in Type 1 diabetes, there may be an initial, transient deterioration in pre-existing retinopathy when a person changes to tight control from a less rigorous insulin regime. Other weapons in the fight against retinopathy include regular specialist screening (retinal eye examination) and, where applicable, laser therapy to treat the condition. These are discussed in greater detail below. The importance of regular eye tests for everyone with diabetes cannot be over-emphasized, especially in the light of the fact that retinopathy usually causes no symptoms until the damage has been done and the condition is quite advanced. There are several recognized stages of retinopathy.

Background Retinopathy
This is the first stage of the condition in which there is early damage to the blood vessels, causing them to enlarge and leak fluids and deposits onto the retina. When the retina is examined, there may be evidence of waxy deposits, minute haemorrhages or aneurysms or a retinal blot, but this stage produces no symptoms. If the background retinopathy is detected, the person is usually monitored closely with further, regular eye screening. The level of glycaemic control may be discussed and intensifying insulin therapy may be an appropriate response. Also, a thorough physical check-up may be recommended in order to identify other possible problems, particularly high blood pressure and evidence of NEPHROPATHY.

Pre-proliferative Retinopathy
This is a more advanced stage, but one which still produces no symptoms. Examination of the eye is likely to

reveal multiple small haemorrhages and 'cotton-wool' spots, along with other abnormalities but there is no formation of new blood vessels. There is a high risk of progression to the next stage of proliferative retinopathy and hence the person will normally be referred to a specialist ophthalmologist for an early appointment. An overall health review, including glycaemic control and checking for other possible complications, may also be recommended.

Proliferative Retinopathy

This is characterized by the growth of new blood vessels in response to growth factors released by parts of the retina that have been starved of their normal blood supply, due to previous damage. These new vessels are very fragile and are subject to bleeding into the vitreous body (the jelly-like layer of the eye). There may be scar tissue formation causing a detachment of the retina, the appearance of 'floaters' (spots travelling across the field of vision), or a sudden painless loss of sight due to a larger haemorrhage into the vitreous body. Proliferative retinopathy threatens sight itself and it most commonly occurs in people with Type 2 diabetes. When detected, an immediate referral to an ophthalmology clinic follows without delay. The eyes are assessed and the person is given laser treatment to selectively destroy the parts of the retina that have been damaged. This halts the response to produce new vessels, while those that have already been formed degenerate without causing further harm. Laser therapy preserves the sight but it cannot restore what has already been lost. Several sessions may be needed to burn all the damaged areas of the retina.

Advanced Diabetic Eye Disease

This is characterized by retinal detachment due to the formation of scar tissue and the growth of new, fragile vessels on the iris (the muscular disc which controls the amount of light that enters the eye through the pupil). There may also be haemorrhages into the vitreous body and the person may notice floaters travelling across the eye. New blood vessel formation on the iris is called rubeosis iridis and it may interfere with the natural drainage of the eye, causing secondary glaucoma which can be painful. A person with this stage of eye disease is in danger of major or complete loss of sight in the affected eye and will already be receiving ophthalmological specialist care. Laser treatment and possibly other microsurgery may be needed to remove fibrous scar tissue plaques and reattach parts of the retina.

Maculopathy

This is more common in people with Type 2 diabetes and three different forms are recognized. The condition is characterized by leakage of fluids from damaged capillaries which builds up in the small area of the retina responsible for central vision called the macula. Usually, the material that is leaked is hard and forms plaques (exudative maculopathy) or rings with fluid at their centre (oedematous maculopathy). There is a gradual loss of visual sharpness leading to considerable deterioration in the person's ability to see. Once again, prompt referral to an ophthalmologist is required and surgical intervention is usually necessary to preserve sight. If there is accompanying HYPERTENSION, additional measures must be taken to reduce this.

Cataracts

Cataracts are five times more likely to occur in people with diabetes and also tend to develop at a younger age than in the non-diabetic population. A rare form of rapidly developing 'snowflake' cataract can occasionally occur in young people with Type 1 diabetes. Its development usually follows a period when glycaemia has been poorly controlled. Cataracts can normally be successfully treated by means of surgery.

Glaucoma

Glaucoma, as a primary condition, is also more likely to occur in people with diabetes and may additionally arise as a secondary complication (rubeosis iridis) of ADVANCED DIABETIC EYE DISEASE. Glaucoma is characterized by high intraocular pressure within the eye, caused by a build-up of fluid when normal drainage is obstructed. It is a sight-threatening condition which often produces no symptoms but can be detected by regular eye testing. Treatment is by means of drops and tablets to reduce the production of the fluid responsible for the build-up of pressure, and possibly surgery to reopen an outlet for drainage of the eye.

Neuropathy (Nerve Damage)

Neuropathy means damage to the nerves and conditions that arise as a result of this damage and it is the most common complication of diabetes. It may affect a single nerve or groups of nerves and has numerous clinical manifestations. Symptoms may be few or absent, especially in the early stages, but some forms of neuropathy cause severe pain and are highly disabling. The cause of diabetic neuropathy is not fully understood, but two, and possibly three, sets of factors are believed to be important. First, hyperglycaemia in diabetes causes increased activation of a biochemical pathway known as the polyol pathway. There is an accumulation of sorbitol and fructose (sugars derived from glucose) within nerves, which interferes with other biochemical reactions and impairs the ability to transmit electrical signals. Secondly, again as a result of hyperglycaemia, the disruption of biochemical pathways is believed to cause damage to blood vessels supplying nerves, possibly starving them of oxygen and nutrients and contributing to the damage seen in neuropathy. Thirdly, other conditions, not directly connected with diabetes, may contribute to the development of neuropathy in some people. Studies have shown that good, and especially 'tight', glycaemic control can greatly reduce the incidence and progression of clinical (i.e. detectable) neuropathy in diabetes.

Sensory nerves carry signals from the sense organs to the brain and are involved in the perception of the senses such as touch and pain. Motor nerves carry signals from the brain and spinal cord to voluntary muscles that move limbs and joints. The autonomic nervous system governs all the unconscious, involuntary functions of the body such as control of the major organs, such as the heart, kidneys, gastrointestinal system, bladder and so on. Neuropathy can affect one or more nerves involved in all these areas of the nervous system and this helps to explain why the manifestations can be so diverse. Several stages in the development and progression of neuropathy are recognized.

1. Biochemical changes within nerves, as in the abnormal build up of sorbitol. Produces no symptoms.
2. Reduced ability of nerves to conduct electrical impulses so that speed of conduction is reduced. May be detected

by electrophysiological measurements but causes no symptoms.

3. Clinical neuropathy, which can be diagnosed using various tests, depending upon the type (*see* CLASSIFICATION OF DIABETIC NEUROPATHY below).

4. Late or end-stage complications in which there is significant damage to nerves and disruption of their function, with surrounding tissues affected. Examples include *ulcers*, *gangrene* and Charcot's foot or CHARCOT NEURO-ARTHROPATHY.

Classification of Diabetic Neuropathy

Since neuropathy manifests itself in such a wide range of forms, it may be classified in somewhat different ways, even by clinicians. However the following clinical classification is in use.

• Localized or focal neuropathies. These affect particular nerves: examples are carpal tunnel syndrome and palsies of the cranial nerves. These conditions also occur in people who do not have diabetes, but less commonly.

• Distal symmetrical polyneuropathy or 'glove and stocking' neuropathy. This condition is the most common form of diabetic neuropathy but it usually does not produce symptoms in the early stage. It tends to progress with the duration of diabetes and may be associated with other diabetic complications. It is a major factor in diabetic foot disease, affecting sensory nerves and sympathetic (autonomic) nerves. Motor nerves may also show abnormalities but this usually does not produce symptoms.

• Acute, diffuse, painful sensory neuropathy. This is an uncommon form which is abrupt in its occurrence and may begin following initial treatment with insulin. It is not related to the length of time the person has had diabetes and is not connected with other diabetic complications. It usually gets better with time, although not always completely.

- Motor neuropathies. These are unusual forms of which the best known example is amyotrophy of Garland (also a form of mononeuropathy). The cause is unknown but recovery may take up to one year and is sometimes incomplete.

- Autonomic neuropathy. This affects the nerves of the autonomic nervous system, which controls many organs and functions within the body. The stomach, intestine, bladder, heart and penis are the organs most likely to be affected. The most common form of this type of neuropathy is erectile dysfunction in men, which may have other contributory causes. It is especially important for older men with diabetes to know that problems of sexual performance are common and well understood. Clinical care staff are trained in this area and effective help is available to men with this problem.

- Diffuse, small fibre neuropathy. This is an unusual and distinctive form of autonomic neuropathy that most commonly occurs in young women with Type 1 diabetes. It is associated with iritis (inflammation of the iris of the eye) and it is believed that it may have an autoimmune cause.

These various types of neuropathy are discussed below in greater detail.

Focal Neuropathies
These may affect certain cranial nerves or peripheral nerves and are thought to be caused by lesions on blood vessels which in turn cause pressure and swelling of nerves.

Carpal tunnel syndrome affects the wrist and hand and is due to compression of the median nerve within the restricted space through which it has to pass. Symptoms include 'pins and needles', numbness, tingling, burning or radiating pain involving upper parts of the arm. Other focal neuropathies may affect the elbow (due to compression of the ulnar nerve) or foot (known as 'foot drop') caused by pressure on the peroneal nerve. Sometimes these conditions resolve with time, but treatment, consisting of injections of certain drugs or surgical decompression of the affected nerve, may be required in severe cases.

Distal Symmetrical Polyneuropathy

This common form of neuropathy most often involves the feet and legs but occasionally, if advanced, the hands may be affected. It is a major contributory cause of diabetic foot disease but may be symptomless, especially in the early stages although the disorder is a progressive one. A range of symptoms and clinical signs may be present:

- feeling of numbness and/or having cold feet
- tingling, 'pins and needles', or odd sensation in the feet that has been likened to walking barefoot on pebbles
- pain, which can be constant, burning or shooting in character
- unpleasant sensitivity to contact with clothing and bed clothes, a condition known as allodynia
- cramp-like pains in the legs, especially occurring in bed at night
- loss of the ability of the feet to sweat
- loss of reflexes (ankle jerks)
- unsteadiness of gait due to reduction in sense of position and balance

- postural hypotension (fall in blood pressure upon rising upright)
- warm, cracked skin on feet
- clawing of the toes.

There are two main ways of dealing with this condition: primary prevention and symptomatic treatment. Primary prevention consists of good or tight glycaemic control which has been shown to preserve and protect nerve function. In people who already have the condition, good control may help to prevent it from worsening but symptoms themselves have to be treated on an individual basis. Various pain-relieving drugs are used which may help, and also a cream, capsaicin (containing an active alkaloid found in hot red peppers), is effective in some people when applied to the skin. Certain tricyclic antidepressants block the neurotransmitter noradrenaline, released by the sympathetic nervous system, and may help to reduce pain, especially when taken with other analgesic drugs.

Anticonvulsants, such as carbamazepine may help to relieve the shooting pains that some people experience. Allodynia occurring at night may be relieved by using a bed cradle to lift the covers off the lower limbs. An alternative is a special film called opsite which, when applied to the skin, acts as a barrier to the stimuli that cause pain, although it is not effective for everyone. People affected by this neuropathy need to be especially vigilant about foot care to avoid a deterioration in the condition (*see* DIABETIC FOOT DISEASE below). Finally, counselling and psychological support are extremely important for this distressing condition, especially reassurance that painful symptoms can be helped and may naturally abate.

Acute, Diffuse, Painful, Sensory Neuropathy
Usually, this form of neuropathy resolves with time and affected people need reassurance that this is likely to occur. In the meantime, symptomatic relief using various drugs and other approaches, as described above, can be offered.

Motor Neuropathies
The best-known example is diabetic neuropathy of Garland, with other forms, such as truncal neuropathy affecting the abdomen, occurring far more rarely. Amyotrophy may arise in Type 1 and Type 2 diabetes, and the affected person is usually male and aged 50 years or older, with Type 2 syndrome. The onset of the condition is rapid, affecting the quadriceps muscle of one or both thighs. There is pain, weakness and muscle wasting which develops rapidly and affects walking and normal activity. There is a typical loss of the normal knee-jerk reflex. Other symptoms include weight loss, insomnia and depression, which means that the psychological impact of amyotrophy can be severe. The cause remains uncertain, but pain and other symptoms usually subside after about three months and the person slowly recovers. However, recovery may take more than a year and although there may be residual muscle wasting, it is not usually severe enough to cause ongoing weakness. Recurrence is uncommon. Treatment consists of introducing good or tight glycaemic control, pain relief, physiotherapy and psychological support and care. Above all, the affected person needs to be reassured that recovery, even though it may be slow, is the expected outcome.

Autonomic Neuropathy
It is believed that 30 to 40 per cent of people with diabetes, particularly those who have had the condition for a long

time, may have signs of autonomic neuropathy which is a form that usually produces symptoms. As mentioned above, erectile dysfunction in men is the most common manifestation and this is discussed below but other symptoms and signs include the following.

Gustatory Sweating

This occurs during eating and in rare cases can be copious and drenching in nature. It is a common symptom and it seems to be triggered especially by eating strongly flavoured food such as cheese. Unfortunately, effective treatment is lacking. Anticholinergic drugs have been tried but are not satisfactory since they may produce side-effects that are more unpleasant than the sweating.

Diarrhoea

Diarrhoea is fortunately an uncommon and intermittent symptom of autonomic neuropathy. It usually occurs interspersed with periods of normal bowel habit or even constipation. It may occur at night and can cause a degree of incontinence and so is very distressing for the person affected. A person suffering from recurrent diarrhoea will need to undergo tests and investigation to rule out other causes such as inflammatory diseases of the bowel. If the cause is autonomic neuropathy, it is believed that the disruption of normal movements of the bowel due to nerve damage allows overgrowth of intestinal bacteria and that it is this that is responsible for the intermittent bouts of diarrhoea. If the cause is bacterial, a good response is often achieved by treatment with courses of antibiotics. Effective drugs, such as codeine phosphate, are available to control diarrhoea.

Gastroparesis

This is another, fortunately uncommon, symptom characterized by bouts of severe vomiting and regurgitation of food. There may also be nausea, bloating, pain and weight loss and if severe, treatment in hospital may be required. Gastroparesis occurs when the vagus nerve, which controls stomach emptying, is affected, and the condition requires careful evaluation and treatment. It may be necessary to give intravenous fluids, and sometimes nutrition via a nasogastric tube, in the first instance, to people who are severely affected. Once the initial symptoms have been stabilized, good glycaemic control will be initiated and various drug treatments are likely to be needed.

Bladder Dysfunction

This occurs when the sacral nerves are affected by neuropathy and the most common symptom is a reduced ability to pass urine. However, neuropathic bladder dysfunction is relatively rare. Incomplete emptying of the bladder leads to an increased risk of infection. Symptoms include a feeling of bladder fullness even after urinating, a poor urine stream and degrees of incontinence. Men with this condition are likely to be impotent. Mechanical methods of emptying the bladder, possibly including the use of a catheter, may be needed and infections are treated with antibiotics. Impotence can also be treated by various methods.

Postural Hypotension

Postural hypotension is low blood pressure on rising from a prone position and it is usually worse at night. Symptoms include dizziness, feelings of weakness and fainting, and the condition requires careful evaluation and treatment with various drugs. It may also be helpful to raise the head end of the bed and to wear elastic support stockings.

Cardiac/Respiratory Arrest

Cardiac/respiratory arrest can occur as a result of autonomic nerve damage affecting the heart. There is an increased risk of heart attack, especially following surgery, if the condition has not been detected. For this reason, people with diabetes who need planned surgery are very carefully monitored before, during and after their operation. Care of those who may be at risk, such as people who are detected with heartbeat abnormalities, is especially rigorous. It is thought that neuropathic, autonomic nerve damage of the heart may be responsible for the rare occurrence of sudden death in young people with Type 1 diabetes.

Erectile Dysfunction and Impotence

Erectile dysfunction and impotence means the inability to sustain an erection for a long enough period of time to achieve sexual intercourse. It may also be called impotence and may be accompanied by a failure to achieve orgasm and ejaculation. Erectile dysfunction at some stage in life is an almost universal male experience, usually as a transitory problem. It becomes increasingly common with advancing age and is particularly likely to affect those with diabetes. It is believed that it may affect 30 per cent of men with diabetes overall, rising to 55 per cent and possibly higher, in those aged over 60. Erectile dysfunction can have several contributory causes, of which autonomic neuropathy is felt to be the most important. Others are peripheral vascular disease, particularly atherosclerosis or narrowing of the arteries supplying the genital organs. A reduced blood supply can affect the ability both to achieve and to maintain an erection. A range of drugs can be a contributory cause, particularly antihypertensives (thiazide diuretics, beta-blockers) and others. These are drugs that may be used to treat conditions connected with diabetes, and so men who are also affected by autonomic nerve damage can be especially vulnerable to erectile dysfunction. A whole range of psychological factors – anxiety, stress, depression, relationship problems – also have an adverse affect. Alcohol and drug abuse are further well-known contributory causes. Less commonly, an existing endocrine disorder may be responsible.

Diabetes clinical care staff and particularly practice nurses, are well aware of the common problem of erectile dysfunction in men affected by diabetes. Many receive specialist training in this area, covering all aspects, including encouraging male patients to talk about the problem. Hence a man reporting this problem will always receive sympathetic help and counselling, along with practical measures to discover the cause and to offer effective treatment. This may involve a detailed physical examination and possible referral to a specialist and an in-depth discussion. The latter is often particularly helpful, especially if the man's partner is involved, in relieving the stress and anxiety which often accompanies the condition. Very often, the most difficult part is to begin to talk about a sexual problem, but once the discussion has occurred most people feel a great sense of relief. There are a number of ways in which the problem can be addressed, depending, first of all upon whether the primary cause is amenable to treatment. Improved glycaemic control is recommended and may help some people, as may changing non-diabetic medications if these are implicated. If reduced blood supply is the problem, drug treatments or surgery can help in some cases. Other drugs, particularly sildenafil (viagra) and mechanical devices such as a vacuum pump are among the other treatment options that are available.

Diffuse Small Fibre Neuropathy

This is a distinctive and unusual form of neuropathy that usually affects young women with Type 1 diabetes. There is severe autonomic nerve damage and CHARCOT NEURO-ARTHROPATHY (*see* below) and it is believed that the cause is autoimmune. The person loses sensation of pain and temperature in the feet or these are greatly reduced. However, the sense of touch and vibration are retained.

Diabetic Foot Disease

Diabetic foot disease involves three elements: peripheral neuropathy (distal symmetrical polyneuropathy), peripheral vascular disease and infection. Neuropathy is usually the principal factor in diabetic foot disease, causing a loss of sensation and disruption of the normal pattern of nerves supplying the muscles of the foot. As a consequence, local areas of high pressure develop due to subtle changes in the internal anatomy of the foot, increasing the risk of the formation of calluses, especially on the 'pad' below the big toe. The neuropathic foot remains warm and the skin is of normal colour (as the blood supply is intact), although it tends to be dry. The foot is highly susceptible to mechanical damage due to loss of sensation, for example from objects that are trodden on and not noticed, or from grit in a shoe, or from inadvertent scalding or burning. Other clinical signs include diminished reflexes and although pain is often absent, this is not invariably the case. If present, the foot is often especially painful at night. People with neuropathic diabetic foot disease are at risk of ulceration on the sole of the foot and, more rarely, CHARCOT ARTHROPATHY.

Peripheral vascular disease relates to disease and damage of the blood vessels supplying outlying areas of the body, in this case, the feet. About half of people with diabetic foot problems have peripheral vascular damage as a contributory cause and may be said to have neuro-ischaemic foot disease. The clinical signs and symptoms of this are somewhat different to those of purely neuropathic foot disease. Sensation in the foot is retained to a greater extent but it tends to feel cold and look pale due to the poor blood supply. Reflexes are retained but pulses are absent, again reflecting the poor blood supply. Calluses are less likely to form but there is a risk of ulcers developing on the extremities of the foot and in extreme cases, gangrene.

Ulcers are one manifestation of the third contributory cause of diabetic foot disease, which is infection. People with neuropathic or neuro-ischaemic foot disease are especially at risk of infection in their feet. In practice, the two types of foot disease are treated and managed in similar ways. However, peripheral vascular disease can occur in the absence of diabetes and known risk factors for its occurrence are smoking, HYPERTENSION and elevated levels of blood cholesterol. All these are of particular significance in diabetes and risks can be reduced by adopting a healthy lifestyle and diet and taking regular EXERCISE.

Overall, ulceration and infection of the feet are the most common reason for hospital admittance in people with diabetes. Unfortunately, people with diabetes are 10 to 15 times more likely to undergo amputation (of one or more toes or, rarely, the whole foot), than the non-diabetic population. However, it must be emphasized that amputation is only ever carried out in extreme circumstances, when other treatments have failed and where there is a risk of non-healing and the spread of infection. Amputation may be needed, for example, if serious lesions or osteomyelitis (infection in the bone) occur repeatedly at the same site and do not heal or respond to antibiotic treatment, or if gangrene has set in.

Since Type 2 diabetes is often not identified until quite a late stage, many people are already at risk of foot complications at the time of diagnosis. For this reason, very great emphasis is placed upon good foot care by diabetes clinical care staff. People with diabetes should receive information and advice on this subject, including access to specialist services such as chiropody, and they may require individually fitted, special shoes. Feet are examined on a regular basis during clinical visits so that potential problems can be identified and protective/preventive measures can be put into place. There is ample evidence that good care can prevent the occurrence of foot problems, even in those who are at risk. For example, the most common cause of ulceration is tight or poorly-fitting shoes and this is entirely avoidable with a little extra care.

General advice on foot care for people with diabetes is as follows.

- Wash feet daily in warm water that does not exceed 37 °C. (It is best to use a thermometer to check the temperature, especially if thermal sensation is impaired.) Only use mild soap and do not soak the feet for more than 10 minutes.
- Dry the feet thoroughly, especially between the toes. Trim nails to the shape of the toe, if required, after bathing (but follow specific advice given by the clinic) when they

are softer and easier to cut. If the skin is very dry, use a moisturizing cream recommended by the diabetes clinic.

- Inspect feet carefully once a day – a long-handled mirror is needed to examine the soles. (Some people may need help with this.) Note any changes, however slight, such as an area of redness which might indicate an early-stage lesion or infection. Seek prompt advice if you think that there may be a problem. Corns, calluses, blisters etc. require special attention and should be dealt with according to clinical advice.
- Wear cotton or wool socks that are a good fit but are not too tight.
- Never walk around the house barefoot but always wear slippers or shoes.
- Check the inside of shoes before putting them on for small stones or grit, etc.
- Choose shoes carefully. They need to have plenty of room, especially in the toe and the uppers should be made of leather. (However, some people find good quality, 'breathable' trainers to be a comfortable alternative.) Shoes need to have firm fastenings – laces, buckles or Velcro™ – so that the feet do not slip about inside. Soles should be thick so that stones that are walked on cannot harm the sole of the foot. New shoes need to be 'worn in' – they should only be worn for brief periods at first to make sure that they fit well and do not rub.
- Feet may swell through the day, especially in hot weather. It is necessary to be aware of this and change them for a larger pair, if necessary.
- If you have 'high risk' feet, do not walk excessively especially if you are not accustomed to walking or if the weather is hot or if you are on holiday.

Treatment of ulcers

If not too severe, ulcers may be treated at an out-patient clinic by means of chiropody, antibiotics (if infection is present) and possibly a plaster cast (with a segment cut out over the ulcer), to relieve pressure and maintain the person's mobility. If the ulcer does not heal or infection persists, the person will need to be admitted to hospital for further treatment. Bed rest aids healing and the ulcer needs to be dressed frequently. Antibiotics may need to be given intravenously. If ischaemia is present, a vascular surgeon may assess whether surgical intervention would be helpful.

Charcot Neuroarthropathy

Charcot neuroarthropathy develops in about 0.5 per cent of diabetic people with neuropathic foot disease. Disruption of the sensory nerve supply and subsequent abnormal pressure loading often leads to injury or undetected fracture. There is an increased blood flow to the damaged area and characteristic softening and resorption of the bone leading to deformity. By this stage, the foot is often painful and swollen (due to fluid collection) and feels hot. There is a high risk of infection and ulceration.

Treatment takes place in hospital and usually involves a period of up to three months of non-weight-bearing. A walking plaster cast or one that is removable is usually chosen for essential mobility but the foot must be rested as much as possible. Any infection present is treated intensively with antibiotics, and drugs to inhibit bone deformity may also be needed. The aim is to stabilize and reduce the degree of foot deformity and to preserve mobility. The affected person will require specially made shoes and particular care is needed when he or she starts to walk again.

Diabetic Nephropathy (Kidney Damage)

Diabetic nephropathy is a progressive and serious disease of the kidneys in which the small blood vessels of these organs become damaged and begin to leak. As a result, a protein called albumin is lost or excreted in the urine in increasing amounts. When the loss is still at a relatively low level (30 to 300 mg/day), the condition is called MICROALBUMINURIA and this is the earliest stage that can be detected by sensitive clinical tests. At a higher level of loss, greater than 300 mg/day, the condition becomes known as proteinuria, a stage that can be detected by urine dipstick (albustix) testing. In fact, five progressive stages of diabetic nephropathy, which overlap with one another, are recognized.

1. Increase in blood plasma flow to kidneys, which may themselves be slightly enlarged. These are sub-clinical signs that are usually reversible with good control of glycaemia. There are no symptoms.
2. Early structural changes to kidneys which may develop after about two years. Again, a sub-clinical stage that does not produce symptoms.
3. Microalbuminuria. Detected either by sensitive radio-immunoassay testing or by measuring albumin/creatinine (a metabolic compound) ratio. Does not produce symptoms but blood pressure is often raised.
4. Proteinuria. Detected by positive albustix (dipstick) testing. This is the stage that is called clinical nephropathy. It is accompanied by high blood pressure and elevated levels of creatinine.
5. End-stage renal failure (ESRF). Kidney failure, requiring continual, ongoing treatment.

Nephropathy can have causes other than diabetes, and diagnosis of microalbuminuria is associated with a higher risk of heart and circulatory disease. In diabetes, microalbuminuria is linked with an increased risk of NEUROPATHY and peripheral vascular disease. In addition, there is a close association between nephropathy and RETINOPATHY. About 66 per cent of people with proliferative retinopathy also have associated nephropathy. High blood pressure is another closely associated risk factor. Nephropathy occurs in about one-third of people with Type 1 diabetes, and, overall, a similar proportion of those with Type 2 syndrome are likewise affected. About one-quarter of white Europeans with Type 2 diabetes are affected by nephropathy but for people of Asian, African, Afro-Caribbean, Native Indian and Japanese descent, the incidence is much higher. Up to half of people in these racial groups are at risk of developing the condition.

A person newly diagnosed with diabetes will be asked to provide a urine sample that is then tested for microalbuminuria. If this is negative, routine testing once a year is considered to be the minimal requirement. If microalbuminuria or proteinuria is detected, more frequent testing, along with treatment, is likely to be necessary. Smoking is a high risk factor for the development of microalbuminuria, as well as for the heart and circulatory disease and hypertension that so often coexist with diabetic nephropathy. Giving up smoking, eating healthily, losing weight if necessary, and taking exercise are all important in helping to prevent the condition from developing. Good, and especially 'tight', glycaemic control, has been shown to be effective in reducing the incidence of kidney disease in diabetes. However, if nephropathy has become established, tight glycaemic control does not appear to have an effect upon its progression.

Certain genetic factors have been identified as being important in the development of diabetic nephropathy and these are the subject of intensive research and study. One of these is called the aldose reductase gene, and another the angiotensin-converting enzyme (ACE) gene. In the future, it may be possible to identify people who carry 'at risk' genetic factors for diabetic nephropathy and to find ways of controlling or switching off their damaging effects. The ACE gene is responsible for the normal occurrence of angiotensin-converting enzyme, which regulates blood pressure by acting to constrict blood vessels, making it harder for blood to flow through. The enzyme has a natural role in controlling blood pressure in normal health, but is unhelpful in the presence of high blood pressure. Drugs called ACE inhibitors, which block the action of the enzyme and thereby reduce high blood pressure, are a recognized treatment for hypertension. However, certain types, e.g. Captopril, Lisinopril, Ramipril, Enalopril and Perindopril, have been found to have an additional protective effect on the kidneys with regard to the occurrence and progression of diabetic nephropathy. ACE inhibitors may now be used as preventives in people with normal blood pressure who are showing signs of microalbuminuria. Their use requires careful monitoring and they can produce side-effects, but they appear to be a useful treatment, especially in Type 1 diabetes.

Microalbuminuria
For a diagnosis of microalbuminuria to be made, more than one sample is tested over a period of consecutive days. People

with Type 1 diabetes detected with microalbuminuria are at a 20 per cent higher risk of eventually developing end-stage renal failure. However, in some people, microalbuminuria may be stable, especially if they have had diabetes for a long time. In others, the micralbuminuria may regress, even without intervention. Treatment for the condition is closely allied with that for diabetes as a whole. Ensuring that there is good glycaemic control, dietary adjustment to lower cholesterol and lipid levels, and weight loss if necessary, are all part of treatment. Drugs to lower plasma lipid levels may be needed. In addition, ACE inhibitors may be prescribed, even in the absence of high blood pressure, to protect kidney function. ACE inhibitors must be avoided during pregnancy and are also unsuitable for those who have sustained damage to the blood vessels of the kidneys. Possible side-effects of the drugs include diarrhoea, nausea, a dry cough, headache, and low blood pressure causing dizziness. Anyone taking these drugs requires regular check-ups, and microalbuminuria needs to be monitored by means of regular urine testing.

Proteinuria
Treatment of the high blood pressure which is established by this stage is considered to be essential as this can slow the rate of progression of the nephropathy. ACE inhibitors, or a number of other drugs, may be prescribed, sometimes in combination. Drugs to lower plasma lipid levels, such as statins, may be needed. In people with Type 1 diabetes, restriction of animal protein in the diet has been found to be helpful. Vegetable protein is believed to be less harmful to the damaged kidneys but dietary changes need to be carefully worked out under the supervision of a dietitian. Since

kidney function is disrupted by this stage, there is a risk of elevated levels of potassium (hyperkalaemia) and a fall in the amount of calcium in the blood. Hence people with proteinuria require ongoing careful monitoring and may need to take a number of different types of drug to support and balance the failing kidneys. People with Type 2 diabetes who have developed proteinuria require insulin treatment. People with clinical nephropathy, the alternative name for proteinuria, require psychological support and counselling to help them to come to terms with impending kidney failure and the probable future need for dialysis.

Nephrotic Syndrome

This is a complication of several kidney disorders, including diabetic nephropathy. In diabetes, it is characterized by heavy proteinuria accompanied by HYPERTENSION and other clinical signs. Often, there is BACKGROUND RETINOPATHY and fluid retention and there may be other urinary tract damage and infection. It is treated intensively in a similar way to proteinuria.

End-stage Renal Failure

This serious condition can only be treated by renal dialysis or kidney transplant. Unfortunately, people with this condition often have other serious complications as well, particularly, severe RETINOPATHY and heart disease and these may complicate treatment. There may be postural hypertension and NEUROPATHY, with damage to the autonomic nervous system, which can make conventional haemodialysis more difficult to carry out. However, haemodialysis remains the mainstay of treatment for end-stage renal failure. An alternative method is called Continuous Ambulatory

Peritoneal Dialysis (CAPD). This avoids rapid changes in volume of fluids, does not require access into a blood vessel (but into the peritoneal cavity) and is suitable for elderly people and those with heart disease. It has the further advantage that insulin for controlling diabetes can be added to the dialysis bag. The main risk of CAPD is infection and peritonitis. For people aged under 65 years, a kidney transplant is the best treatment option but this is limited by a severe shortage of donor organs. In the USA, organ donation from a living relative is sometimes performed but this is rare in the UK, at least at the present time. The survival rate among transplant patients with diabetes is slightly lower than in those without the condition but this can be a very successful form of treatment for suitable patients. In patients with Type 1 diabetes, a combined pancreas (or part pancreas) and kidney transplant is sometimes (although rarely) performed.

9

LONG-TERM CHRONIC COMPLICATIONS: MACROVASCULAR DISEASES

Macrovascular complications include serious conditions such as heart attack, angina, cardiovascular disease and peripheral vascular disease. Complications vary in occurrence and in progression between the two main type of diabetes. Their incidence is not inevitable and there are individual differences in susceptibility between different people. Environmental and lifestyle factors are known to have an influence. Although macrovascular complications present a risk to people with diabetes, it is important to realize that there are many ways in which this can be reduced, for example, by adopting a healthy diet and lifestyle, maintaining good glycaemic control and refraining from smoking.

Macrovascular disease damages the arteries supplying the heart, brain and legs, increasing the risk of coronary heart disease, such as angina and heart attack, stroke, and peripheral vascular disease (a major contributor to DIABETIC FOOT DISEASE). Macrovascular disease is caused by atherosclerosis (or atheroma), a degenerative disease of the arteries in which the inner walls become scarred, allowing fat deposits to build up, leading to reduced blood flow and narrowing of the vessels. Atherosclerosis and macrovascular disease are major causes of premature death and disability among the general population, as well as in those with diabetes. The risks of developing atherosclerosis increase with eating an unhealthy diet high in saturated fat and salt, obesity, lack of exercise, smoking, HYPERTENSION, and dyslipidaemia (abnormal lipid/cholesterol levels in the blood).

General Treatment and Prevention

The usual methods of healthy eating and diet adjustment to lower the intake of saturated fat, coupled with weight loss if required, and increased exercise, are vitally important for people with diabetes. These measures on their own have been shown to have a beneficial effect upon diabetic HYPERTENSION and dyslipidaemia and thereby to increase life expectancy. As previously noted, hypertension is particularly common among the majority of people, those with Type 2 syndrome, and is also associated with insulin resistance in this group. In Type 1 diabetes, it is mainly associated with the occurrence of diabetic nephropathy. Hypertension is a major risk factor for macrovascular complications (as well as microvascular ones) and bringing it under control is therefore of great importance, both for these reasons and for the general management of diabetes. Along with lifestyle measures, a variety of drugs are used, quite often in combination, as has already been seen.

Diabetic dyslipidaemia is particularly common in Type 2 diabetes, and when it occurs in Type 1 disease it is especially associated with NEPHROPATHY. Once again, dietary measures and cholesterol- and lipid-lowering drugs such as statins may be used in treatment.

Stopping smoking, if applicable, is probably the most important immediate way to lessen the risk of macrovascular complications, both in people with diabetes and in those who are not affected by the condition.

At the diabetes clinic, regular checks should be made on cholesterol and lipid levels, carried out at least once a year or more often if necessary. Blood pressure is also routinely monitored and patients are encouraged to follow a healthy diet and lifestyle. All these measures are beneficial for diabetes as a whole as well as being protective with regard to macrovascular disease. People who are considered to be at particular risk of macrovascular complications may be advised to take a small daily dose of enteric-coated aspirin, which thins the blood and has been shown to be helpful in preventing the formation of clots that can pose a risk of serious episodes such as pulmonary embolism. The more serious macrovascular complications and their treatment are described below.

Coronary Heart Disease

Coronary heart disease is the most common cause of death in people with diabetes. The incidence is two to three times greater in men and four to five times higher in women, compared to the non-diabetic population. Women with diabetes lose the pre-menopausal protection against heart disease that exists in those who do not have the condition. People of South Asian origin who have diabetes are at particularly high risk of developing heart disease. Unfortunately, due to the 'silent' nature of Type 2 diabetes, many people have already sustained atherosclerotic damage and are therefore at increased risk by the time of diagnosis. In people with NEUROPATHY, the painful symptoms of angina or even heart attack may be masked and reduced because of nerve damage. Additionally, there is some evidence that heart disease may develop at a faster rate in people with diabetes and this is why such preventive measures as those described above are considered to be so important. In the immediate aftermath of a heart attack, people with diabetes are at greater risk than those not affected by the condition. In addition to analgesics, drugs which may be used include beta-blockers, thrombolytics, ACE inhibitors and aspirin. A daily dose of enteric-coated aspirin may be recommended following recovery to prevent a recurrence and other heart drugs may also be required.

Stroke
People with diabetes have one and a half to two times greater risk of a stroke than the general population. Afro-Caribbean people appear to be at a particular risk. Treatment of a stroke is the same, whether diabetes is present or not. It involves intensive care and monitoring with the use of a variety of different drugs. Once the immediate danger is past, there follows a period of recovery and rehabilitation, involving physiotherapy, occupational therapy and possibly speech therapy, which may be quite prolonged. Disability following a stroke may mean that the person with diabetes requires ongoing help in order to manage their condition.

Peripheral Vascular Disease
This disease is twice as likely to occur in people with diabetes and is a major contributor to DIABETIC FOOT DISEASE. Risk factors for its development include smoking, HYPERTENSION and lipid abnormalities and it principally affects the circulation to the lower limbs and feet. It contributes to the development of ulcers in about half of all patients with diabetic foot lesions and its existence can impede

healing. Peripheral vascular disease has a typical pattern of clinical signs and is diagnosed by a number of different techniques. Appropriate and vigilant foot care, drug treatments (aspirin and vasodilators to improve blood flow) and surgery are used to manage and treat the condition. Preventative measures are the same as those used for other forms of macrovascular disease.

10

DIABETES IN PREGNANT WOMEN, CHILDREN, THE ELDERLY AND ETHNIC MINORITY GROUPS

Diabetes and Pregnancy

Diabetes during pregnancy can take several different forms. Type 1 or Type 2 diabetes may be already present and recognized, and this may be easier to deal with, in that planning and preparations for the pregnancy can begin before conception. Also, the woman is already used to dealing with her diabetes and so is not faced with the possible psychological or emotional impact of a new diagnosis. However, GESTATIONAL DIABETES, in which forms of the syndrome are diagnosed during pregnancy, is quite common (*see also* Chapter 1, GESTATIONAL DIABETES MELLITUS). In some cases, the diabetes (usually Type 2) was pre-existing but had not been diagnosed and is 'unmasked' by the physiological changes that occur. In other cases, diabetic conditions are precipitated by the pro-diabetic, physiological changes of pregnancy, but glycaemia returns to normal after the birth. However, in the latter case, there is a significant risk (about 30 per cent) of the eventual development of Type 2 diabetes. Studies indicate that this risk can be cut in half if the woman maintains her weight within the ideal range in the future.

Metabolic Changes during Normal Pregnancy

As mentioned above, the metabolic changes that occur during pregnancy have the net effect of being pro-diabetic and this helps to explain why gestational diabetes may arise. These can be briefly summarized as follows:

- decreased sensitivity to insulin
- increased lipolysis, i.e. breakdown of fats to provide glucose.

These changes build up gradually and are most marked after the first three months of pregnancy, with the result that a state of relative INSULIN RESISTANCE develops.

Gestational Diabetes

Transient gestational diabetes usually appears during the last six months of pregnancy and takes the form of either IMPAIRED GLUCOSE TOLERANCE or diabetes. IGT may be suspected if a random reading of fasting plasma glucose between 6 and 8 mmol/l is obtained. Diabetes may be suspected if a random fasting plasma glucose reading greater than 8 mmol/l is obtained. However, diagnosis depends upon a 75 g Oral Glucose Tolerance Test being performed. IGT is then diagnosed if a glucose reading between 9 and 11 mmol/l is obtained, two hours after the glucose challenge. Diabetes is diagnosed if the reading is greater than 11 mmol/l. There are a number of risk factors for the development of gestational diabetes. These include:

- being overweight or obese and excessive weight gain during pregnancy
- older mother
- previous glucose intolerance
- previous birth of large baby
- belonging to a high-risk ethnic group

- previous history of hydramnios, an abnormal condition during pregnancy in which an excess quantity of amniotic fluid is produced
- previous glycosuria during pregnancy on two or more separate times of testing.

Screening for gestational diabetes takes the form of periodic testing of urine for the presence of glucose and also blood testing, at the first ante-natal visit and then repeated between 24 and 28 weeks into the pregnancy. If there are any indications of diabetes, an OGGT will be carried out to confirm the diagnosis. In obese women or those who are gaining a lot of weight, calorie restriction will be suggested and may be sufficient to control IGT in pregnancy. However, 30 per cent of women with gestational diabetes need insulin to control their condition. ORAL ANTIDIABETIC DRUGS are not a recommended treatment during pregnancy. A woman with insulin-treated gestational diabetes requires special care during labour and the birth may need to be induced at 38 to 39 weeks if it has not taken place naturally. Normal delivery is usually possible but since there is an increased likelihood of an extra large baby (macrosomia), a caesarean section may be required. After delivery, all but a small proportion (fewer than 10 per cent) of mothers who have gestational diabetes revert to glucose tolerance within the normal range. Insulin is usually stopped soon after the birth. An OGGT is generally carried out at the six week post-natal check up to ensure that diabetes has resolved. Affected women are advised on the importance of weight control, diet, exercise, and so on, in order to lessen the risk of development of Type 2 diabetes.

Pre-existing Diabetes and Pregnancy

Diabetes is associated with greater risks during pregnancy, particularly for the developing foetus but also for the mother. The good news is that with careful preparation, which should begin before conception, and modern high standards of care, over 90 per cent of diabetic pregnancies result in the birth of a healthy child. Similarly, the great majority of diabetic mothers sustain no harm as a result of pregnancy and childbirth. There are foetal and maternal risks (listed below), but they should not be a cause of alarm but rather regarded as the reasons why extra care is needed and worthwhile.

Risks to Baby

- Incidence of congenital abnormalities increased by a factor of 3 to 4. Good glycaemic control lessens the risk; poor glycaemic control increases the risk tenfold or higher.
- Greater incidence of foetal death, some of which may be connected with congenital abnormalities and poor glycaemic control.
- Greater incidence of complications immediately after birth, especially macrosomia, HYPOGLYCAEMIA, respiratory distress syndrome, jaundice, birth trauma.
- Increased risk of diabetes developing in child.

Risks to Mother

- Greater risk of infection of the urinary tract.
- Greater risk of pre-eclampsia (the development of high blood pressure and fluid retention which requires monitoring and treatment). The risk is 10 per cent in diabetic mothers compared to 4 per cent in those who do not have the condition.

- Deterioration in glycaemic control, especially during the last six months of pregnancy, requiring higher insulin doses (Type 1 diabetes). Type 2 diabetes, previously managed by diet and/or tablets, usually requires insulin therapy.
- Greater rate of lipolysis increases the risk of ketosis and DIABETIC KETOACIDOSIS in women with Type 1 diabetes. However, this is still uncommon.
- Severe morning sickness is a particular problem, especially for women with Type 1 syndrome. Repeated vomiting and inability to eat may lead to ketosis. Ketones must be monitored and anti-sickness drugs may be needed. Severe morning sickness may require hospital treatment so that fluids etc. can be delivered by an intravenous drip.
- Diabetic COMPLICATIONS, especially RETINOPATHY and NEPHROPATHY, can deteriorate during pregnancy, especially if advanced. Women with these conditions require particular care.

Preparations for pregnancy should begin before conception. This takes the form of a full medical check-up and assessment of diabetes and glycaemic control. Good control of glycaemia needs to be in place and the woman should begin to take folic acid supplements to protect the foetus from neural tube defects. It is a good idea to lose weight, if you need to, before becoming pregnant and to make sure that you are eating a healthy, nutritious diet. The status of any existing diabetic complications needs to be assessed. RETINOPATHY may need to be stabilized before conception is attempted and advanced NEPHROPATHY is, sadly, a reason for avoiding pregnancy since the risks to

171

the woman are too great. Obviously, you should not smoke and it is best to give up alcohol as well, especially while trying to conceive and in the early stages of pregnancy. Rubella (German measles) immunity should be checked so that vaccination can be given if required.

Following conception and confirmation of pregnancy, women should attend for a check-up every two weeks, preferably at a special diabetic antenatal clinic. All the usual ante-natal checks are carried out but in addition, blood glucose levels and HBA1c are carefully monitored. The aim is to achieve a normal level of blood sugar throughout the course of the pregnancy, as this reduces the risks to mother and child. Of course, this involves frequent and careful self-monitoring at home, but most pregnant women are highly motivated and readily take this in their stride, even during the miseries of morning sickness! Frequent antenatal visits ensure that potential problems are identified early on and the result of this is that most women enjoy a successful and trouble-free pregnancy.

As noted above, insulin therapy is usually needed during pregnancy, whatever the previous treatment method, and in Type 1 diabetes doses will almost certainly need to be increased. Unfortunately, tight control of glycaemia leads to a greater incidence of severe hypos and some women further experience a loss of hypoglycaemic awareness during pregnancy. Hence it is vital that those closely connected with the woman are involved and know how to help her, should the need arise. The woman herself should take extra care to minimize the risk of hypos by observing the recommended precautions, and if attacks have been occurring it is advisable to avoid driving long distances or spending too much time alone. Fortunately, although hypos are distressing for the person who experiences them, there is no evidence that they are in any way harmful to the baby.

Labour and Delivery

Modern practice is to allow a diabetic pregnancy to proceed to 39 weeks in the absence of any contraindications and then to induce labour in hospital. Home birth is not a safe option for a mother with diabetes. It is safer for both mother and child if the pregnancy does not go beyond full-term and for labour and delivery to be planned. This may mean that labour has to be induced. The woman requires careful monitoring of her diabetes, as well as of the progress of labour and will need to be given insulin and dextrose intravenously. Some women may require a caesarean section, either pre-planned or as a result of events during labour. Following the birth and delivery of the placenta, the mother's insulin requirements return immediately to pre-pregnancy levels. Her blood glucose levels require monitoring but the usual injection regime is normally reinstated as soon as possible.

The baby receives the usual check-up and care given to all newborn infants. Breast-feeding is the best option for both mother and child and the presence of diabetes is no barrier to this. If all is well, the mother with diabetes can soon return home and there is no reason to expect a longer than normal stay in hospital.

Diabetes in Children

For reasons that are not clear, the incidence of childhood diabetes has been rising in recent years, not only in the UK but in many other countries as well. In the UK alone, about 20,000 children have diabetes with around 2,000 new cases being diagnosed each year. In almost all cases, the type involved is autoimmune Type 1 diabetes requiring insulin treatment. However, the high and rising incidence of obesity among Western children has meant that cases of Type 2 diabetes are now occurring, even among this young age group. Much more rarely, the type of diabetes known as MODY (MATURITY ONSET DIABETES OF THE YOUNG, *see* Chapter 1) may affect children, and this possibility has to be kept in mind at the time of diagnosis.

In children, symptoms are usually clear-cut and arise quickly in a matter of weeks or even days. About 25 per cent of children present with DIABETIC KETOACIDOSIS (DKA) and in any event suspicion or diagnosis of diabetes in a child necessitates hospital admission. Often, a short stay in hospital is all that is necessary to initiate insulin therapy. However, the child and his or her family may require a great deal of help and support to overcome the shock of diagnosis, to answer their questions and address their worries and generally to begin to learn about diabetes. If the child is very young, it is often the parents who require the greatest degree of support. Feelings of guilt and anxiety for the child's future health are common and entirely understandable. Parents may also worry that diabetes may occur in their other children or in any future offspring. HYPOGLYCAEMIA is a particular cause for concern and is common in insulin-treated children. Sometimes, especially in young children, the symptoms can be hard to recognize and repeated severe episodes can cause neuropsychological damage. Obviously, this is a considerable potential source of worry for parents, who can suddenly find themselves in the position of being the people mainly responsible for the recognition and treatment of hypoglycaemia. Clear instructions about what to do are vital and it is important to convince parents that an occasional attack, even if severe, will not cause lasting harm to their child.

Very young children require adult assistance to administer insulin. However, older children usually quickly learn to take charge of their own treatment, with support from their parents. Many children are able to take diabetes in their stride and carry on with life in the same way as before. It is very important that they should be encouraged to do this and that diabetes is not seen as a barrier to any normal activity, either at school or in the social environment. The child's teachers need to be informed about the diabetes and the possibility of hypos. Most schools and teachers now have a much better understanding of the condition than in the past.

It is in the teenage years that diabetes may cause the greatest number of problems. Hormonal changes at puberty with their accompanying spurts of growth can disrupt glycaemic control and increase insulin requirements. The young person may have more frequent hypos, which may happen at school, and may be subject to teasing, just at the time when he or she most desperately needs to feel the same as everyone else. Even when understanding and empathy is good, diabetes can be a cause of depression in the teenage years. Like others in their age group, young people with diabetes are not exempt from more serious psychological problems such as eating disorders, which pose a particular danger to their health and wellbeing. In diabetes, a manifestation of this can be missing out insulin doses as a perceived means of losing weight. This may be attempted particularly by teen-age girls and is a problem that is now beginning to be more widely recognized. Fortunately, DIABETIC COMPLICATIONS as such are rare among children and young people.

It is considered to be ideal if children and young people can attend clinics that are specially geared to their own age group, although this is not possible in all areas. However, clinical care staff recognize that it is the affected child who must be listened to and whose opinions must be taken into account in discussions about treatment or problems connected with diabetes. They endeavour to treat each child with sympathy, tact and discretion and to respect confidences, so that a relationship of trust is built up. In this way, it is hoped that the older child or teenager will feel able to discuss problems with the diabetes clinical care team, even if he or she is not confiding in parents or teachers.

Diabetes in the Elderly

Diabetes in the elderly can present particular problems of care, and in general these increase with advancing age. As with the rest of the adult population, most diabetes in this age group is Type 2, and over half of people affected by this form of the syndrome are aged over 60. Symptoms can be vague in older people and it is suspected that many cases go undiagnosed. Also, elderly people often have established COMPLICATIONS, which can sometimes be quite severe, at the time of diagnosis. DIABETIC FOOT DISEASE is particularly common. Elderly people are at greater risk of severe HYPOGLYCAEMIA, which can prove fatal. For this reason, strict control of glycaemia is usually not the best option for this age group. There can be many problems affecting the management of diabetes in the elderly and choice of treatment has to be very carefully assessed on an individual basis. Problems include coexisting medical conditions and complications, intellectual impairment which may make it difficult for the person to understand the nature of diabetes and its treatment, psychological disorders and depression, and social isolation. Sometimes, especially if the person lives alone, the best course of treatment from a medical point of view cannot be implemented and a compromise needs to be reached. Arthritis causes many problems in the management of diabetes although devices have been developed to help overcome some of these, for example to make it easier to inject insulin and monitor blood glucose. Ideally, elderly people should receive plenty of home support from family and friends, as well as from healthcare professionals, and should have ready access to specialist services such as chiropody. Unfortunately, for many, the level of support is far from ideal due in part to the pressure on the Health Service and the fact that many elderly people live alone. However, voluntary organizations including local branches of Diabetes UK are often able to provide some support and help.

Diabetes in People from Ethnic Minority Groups

As has been previously noted, the prevalence of diabetes is generally greater in people of African and Asian origin and this is particularly true of Type 2 syndrome. Also, the diabetes tends to occur at a younger age, and in general there is a quicker progression to a requirement for insulin treatment. There are a number of potential difficulties that can affect the treatment and management of diabetes in people from ethnic minorities. These include diet (some traditional foods are high in fat, sugar and salt), religious customs and cultural beliefs, health beliefs and attitudes, language, and family and social constraints. Among the older generation, understanding of the English language may be limited and this can present difficulties in education about diabetes. It is still the case that most of the information leaflets and educational materials are written in English, with a cultural bias towards the majority population, although the position is now changing, especially in areas where there are large numbers of people from ethnic minorities. Ideally, a diabetes clinic should be able to call upon the services of an independent interpreter in the language required. However, in practice, the interpreter is usually a younger member of the patient's family. This in itself can cause problems with regard to confidentiality, and information may not always be accurately passed on. It is recognized that a person from an ethnic minority may be subject to greater religious, cultural and family constraints and less free to act independently. Hence any suggested dietary and lifestyle changes have to reflect and fit in with this – for example, it is important that the person who prepares the family meals understands the needs of the person with diabetes. Treatment regimes and advice may need to allow for religious customs such as fasting, and compromise may often be needed to allow for religious observance while at the same time safeguarding the person's health.

GESTATIONAL DIABETES has a higher incidence among women from certain racial groups and NEPHROPATHY, CORONARY HEART DISEASE and circulatory disease are common

COMPLICATIONS among people of both sexes. People of Indian origin may have a lower incidence of RETINOPATHY and DIABETIC FOOT DISEASE. Among diabetes healthcare professionals, there is now a greater understanding of the potential difficulties that can occur and a willingness to address these when they arise.

11

LIVING WITH DIABETES

Psychological Aspects of Diabetes

It is beyond the scope of this book to describe all the complexities and possible manifestations of the psychological aspects of diabetes and so the following is an overview of factors that are generally well known and recognized. As can be readily appreciated, diabetes impinges on everyday life to an even greater extent than most other chronic diseases. Managing the condition makes certain demands upon daily life and these change with time and are affected by normal life events. This means that diabetes may not only have a psychological/emotional impact at the time of diagnosis but also ongoing, long-lasting effects which can all too easily be overlooked. Diabetes clinical care staff are well aware of the psychological effects of diabetes and are trained both to help directly and to recognize more complex conditions that require referral to a specialist.

The way in which a person comes to terms with diabetes, both at the time of diagnosis and in the longer term, depends upon an enormous range of different factors which include the following:

- personality and temperament – general outlook on life
- general health beliefs as well as specific ones concerning diabetes (e.g. does the person believe that he or she can positively influence/alter health outcomes through his or her actions?)
- type of diabetes and method of treatment required
- presence or absence of diabetic complications

- presence or absence of other diseases, conditions or disabilities
- presence or absence of existing psychological problems or illness
- religious/philosophical beliefs
- level of family and social support
- age – children, young people and the elderly may experience particular difficulties
- occupation (is diabetes likely to affect the person's present or future employment/career prospects?)
- ambitions (does diabetes prevent the person from achieving cherished goals in life, e.g. in sport, or does the person believe that it may do so in the future?).

These are just some of the factors that influence people's responses to diabetes, both at the time of diagnosis and as time progresses. Reaction to the diagnosis may be one of relief, especially if adverse symptoms have been experienced that are readily corrected with the instigation of treatment. In contrast, others may deny the diagnosis or become angry and depressed, especially if they have only negative beliefs about diabetes. Parents of a newly diagnosed child often feel totally misplaced guilt. Sometimes people pass through a series of stages, similar to the process of grieving, before they are able to come to terms with the diagnosis. These may include denial, anger, bargaining, sorrow, and finally acceptance. There may be continuing sorrow at the loss of spontaneity/freedom of action imposed by diabetes which is likely to manifest itself as depression. Indeed, it is recognized that there is both a higher incidence and risk of depression among people with diabetes, especially among those who develop complications. However, there are many people who are bravely stoical, even in the face of painful or disabling complications. Following diagnosis, some people become over-anxious about controlling their diabetes, almost to an obsessional extent. This usually expresses itself in frequent blood and urine testing, inflexibility in type of food eaten, with meal times, exercise and other activities planned down to the smallest detail. If clinical care staff suspect that diabetes is taking over someone's life to this extent, they try to help the person to achieve a more relaxed and balanced view.

In time, most people come to terms with their diabetes, adjust to the demands that it imposes and get on with leading a normal life. Obviously, this is more likely to occur if they are free from complications and have caring family and social support. It also happens more rapidly and is more likely to occur when people receive information that they can understand clearly, along with support, guidance and encouragement in managing their diabetes. This is a further reason why education and the whole concept of 'empowering' people to manage their diabetes and to help themselves, are considered to be so important.

However, it is recognized that psychological problems, particularly depression, are an ever-present threat, even among those who normally cope well. Most people experience mild depression at some stage in life, usually for some entirely understandable reason. Loss of a job and unemployment, leaving home, bereavement, marriage breakdown, accident, illness and innumerable other stressful situations, affecting either oneself or a loved one, are all causes of depression. In someone with diabetes, stress can have the added effect of playing havoc with glycaemic control, giving the person an additional problem to deal with. Factors directly connected with diabetes can themselves be a cause of depression. These can be wide-ranging and include always having to carry diabetes equipment, HBGM, insulin injections, being overweight and finding it difficult to lose weight, impotence for which no help has been sought, and hypos. With hypos, it is not only the episodes themselves that can be a cause of depression but fear of the social consequences and embarrassment of having a public attack. People worry about the odd behaviour that they may exhibit and that this may be misunderstood, or that they will be exposed to ridicule. Young people especially may have particular worries about the social effects of hypos, unfortunately not without foundation. There can be a woeful lack of understanding about diabetes and hypos in schools, and school friends and even teachers can be unsympathetic, although this situation is fortunately not as common as it was in the past. In the worst cases, fears and depression can result in a young person refusing to attend school or engage in social activities, and in this situation professional help is required.

In all these circumstances, the support and advice of diabetes clinical care staff is invaluable. Even if the problem causing the stress and depression cannot be removed altogether, it can almost certainly be diminished in its impact and strategies can be worked out to help the person cope. The diabetes clinic is the obvious first port of call for anyone with the condition who is suffering from psychological problems. Diabetes UK is also a vital source of help and has local branches throughout the country or can be contacted via the Internet.

Many aspects of daily living with diabetes have already been discussed in previous chapters. In this chapter, a few new topics are introduced which have not been covered elsewhere.

Exercise

Exercise is good for everyone, whether they have diabetes or not, and this is particularly the case in modern Britain, at a time when lifestyles have become increasingly sedentary and more people than ever are either overweight or obese. The benefits of taking regular exercise include:

- strengthening the heart (and circulation) to pump blood more efficiently and reduce the risk of heart and circulatory disease
- lowering effect upon blood pressure
- burning up calories, helping in regulation of weight
- strengthening bones and reducing the risk of osteoporosis in later life
- reducing risk of some other conditions including haemorrhoids, constipation and cancer of the colon
- maintaining joint flexibility, especially important in later life.

For people with diabetes, there are additional potential benefits, especially with more intense physical exercise. These include increased insulin sensitivity in muscles and the liver which can result in a reduction in the dose of oral hypoglycaemic drugs or insulin that the person requires. Also, lipid profiles tend to improve. More specifically, helpful HDL cholesterol levels increase and there may be an overall decline in triglycerides, reducing the risk of atherosclerosis. It is thought that lack of exercise may be a direct risk factor for the development of INSULIN RESISTANCE in Type 2 diabetes, and remaining physically active throughout life is one means of protection and prevention.

The Health Education Authority recommends that everyone should aim for half an hour of moderate exercise on at least five days each week. Moderate exercise includes brisk walking, swimming, aerobics, dancing, cycling, team sports, jogging etc., but many other activities can contribute as well. They include active gardening, housework or DIY, running up a flight of stairs or chasing after an active toddler! The advice to all who are about to embark upon a programme of exercise, especially if previously inactive, is the same. This is to start slowly and gently and gradually build up your level of exercise, as and when you become fitter. People with diabetes need to take extra care but the extent of this varies with their age, the type of diabetes and the way it is being treated and the nature of the exercise. General advice is as follows.

• Seek expert advice from your diabetes clinic or general practitioner before undertaking any exercise programme. A medical check-up may be needed if vigorous exercise is contemplated and is always necessary for middle-aged and elderly people. The principal risk is from a cardiovascular event brought on by unaccustomed strenuous exercise.
• Always build up the amount of exercise gradually, over a period of weeks.
• Do not launch straight into strenuous exercise, even if you believe that you are fit.
• Spend ten minutes at the start and end of the exercise period doing gentle stretching, bending, flexing etc. so that your muscles are prepared.
• Use appropriate, good quality sports clothing, footwear, helmet etc. Be especially careful about taking care of your feet.
• Do not exercise during periods when glycaemic control is erratic or poor.

- Do not exercise when you have an illness or infection, however mild.
- Avoid exercise in very hot weather.
- Monitor blood glucose before, during and after exercise, as advised by your diabetes care team.
- Adjust insulin/sulphonylurea doses and/or eat extra carbohydrate-containing snacks, as necessary (*see* below).
- Drink lots of sugar-free fluids before and during the exercise period to avoid dehydration.

In order to understand the need for extra care during exercise if you have diabetes, it is useful to look at what happens in normal health. If exercise is vigorous and continues for more than a few minutes, muscle glycogen stores are broken down and used in the first instance, and circulating glucose and non-esterified fatty acids are utilized. In the liver, the process of glyconeogenesis begins and increases to provide more glucose energy. At the same time, insulin levels fall and counter-regulatory hormones promote mobilization of liver and fat cell energy stores. The system is very finely tuned but if exercise is prolonged for several hours, HYPOGLYCAEMIA will normally occur unless the person eats a carbohydrate-containing meal. The person is not likely to be able to continue to exercise unless energy supplies are restored. In people with diabetes, the normal regulatory mechanisms are impaired and there is the presence of injected insulin or oral antidiabetic drugs which further complicate the metabolic relationships during exercise.

Exercise and Type 1 Diabetes
The effects of exercise on those with Type 1 diabetes depends upon a number of different factors:

- the degree of glycaemic control
- the amount and type of the last insulin dose injected before exercise
- the timing of the last injection and carbohydrate-containing snack or meal in relation to the time of exercise
- the type of exercise and the length of time for which it is performed
- the position of the injection site.

The Degree of Glycaemic Control

If glycaemic control is good, a fall in blood glucose levels occurs due to the energy demands of exercise, in the presence of full insulinization. Exogenous or externally delivered insulin cannot be got rid of (as is the case in normal health) and so there is hyperinsulinaemia while glucose is being used up. The presence of insulin both inhibits glucose production in the liver and the utilization of lipids to provide energy. In these circumstances, HYPOGLYCAEMIA is the likely result, unless the insulin dose and/or carbohydrate intake are altered (*see* below). If glycaemic control is less good or inadequate, there may be a relative state of hypoinsulinaemia before exercise is undertaken. In these circumstances, as glucose is used up during exercise, liver production of glucose increases, counter-regulatory hormones are mobilized and lipids are utilized. The uptake of glucose by muscles is inhibited and the net result is that blood glucose levels rise and there is hyperglycaemia. There is a likelihood of liver ketogenesis, with ketones being produced, and ketonuria.

The Nature of the Insulin Dose

The nature of the insulin dose given before exercise affects the timing of the HYPOGLYCAEMIA that is likely to occur.

A short-acting insulin dose may reach a peak of maximum effect during the exercise period and cause hypoglycaemia, unless sufficient carbohydrate is eaten and/or the dose has been reduced. Longer-acting insulin maintains a high level of insulin in peripheral tissues and has a more prolonged effect, and so hypoglycaemia is more likely to occur several hours after the exercise period, or even during the following day. This means that it is important to eat carbohydrate-containing meals and snacks as usual, to counteract this effect.

The importance of the Timing of the Insulin Dose and Carbohydrate Intake

The timing of both insulin dose and carbohydrate intake in relation to that of exercise are important in preventing or reducing the risk of problems. Ideally, exercise should be planned and carried out one to two hours after a meal. Planned vigorous exercise should be timed to avoid the peak of activity of the last insulin dose.

The Type of Exercise

Vigorous and/or prolonged exercise makes greater demands on the body and its metabolic activity and hence is more likely to cause problems. It requires a greater degree of forward planning, in particular a reduction in the previous insulin dose of 40 to 50 per cent and extra carbohydrate, at a rate of 20 to 40 g per hour, during the exercise period. However, you should seek specific clinical advice.

The Position of the Injection Site

The injection site affects the rate at which insulin is absorbed and hence the time in which it begins to take effect.

It is absorbed at a faster rate from a limb that is being exercised and so it may be advisable to inject into the abdomen. Regardless of the injection site, the effect of exercise is to speed up absorption and hence action of insulin.

Exercise Advice for those with Type 1 Diabetes

Adjustment to exercise depends upon individual factors and each person with Type 1 diabetes should seek advice from the diabetes clinic. It is only possible to give general advice here.

- If the exercise is gentle, there is probably no need to adjust either insulin dose or carbohydrate intake, but monitor blood glucose levels carefully.
- If the exercise is unplanned, more active or carried out for a relatively short period, you may need to eat a carbohydrate-containing snack during and after carrying it out. Monitor blood glucose levels carefully.
- Plan ahead if the exercise is to be active and/or prolonged. Reduce the pre-exercise insulin dose, according to clinical advice and monitor blood glucose levels before, during and after exercise and note the results. Begin the exercise 1 to 2 hours after eating a meal and have suitable carbohydrate snacks and drinks with you that you can take when needed. Ideally, always exercise at the same time of day so that it is easier to monitor the effects of adjusting the insulin dose/carbohydrate intake and to know what you need to do to avoid problems.
- Even if blood glucose levels are high after exercise, do not miss out normal meals and snacks that you eat at regular times. HYPOGLYCAEMIA can still occur in these circumstances, often many hours later as glucose stores used up during exercise are replenished. Refraining

from eating only increases the risk.
- Never omit an insulin dose.
- Due to the risk of hypoglycaemia, some dangerous sports are ill-advised, particularly if undertaken alone. The governing bodies of certain sports (some forms of motor racing, scuba diving, solo sailing, hang-gliding), prohibit participation by insulin-treated people. Diabetes UK is able to advise on the nature of any restrictions that may apply to particular sports.

Exercise and Type 2 Diabetes

People with Type 2 diabetes may retain the normal physiological responses to exercise but to a lesser or altered degree. There is generally no risk of HYPOGLYCAEMIA, except for those being treated with insulin or SULPHONYLUREAS. Those receiving insulin treatment need to observe the same precautions as people with Type 1 diabetes. If treatment is by means of sulphonylureas, the action that is required depends, once again, upon a combination of factors, which include the nature and duration of the exercise and mode of action of the drug, degree of glycaemic control, body weight and individual responses. Expert advice should sought as to whether drug doses need to be altered, and as in Type 1 diabetes it is best to pre-plan any exercise that is strenuous and/or of long duration. It is usually preferable to reduce (or possibly even omit) the pre-exercise sulphonylurea to lessen the risk of hypoglycaemia, rather than increase carbohydrate intake, simply because there may be a need to lose weight. However, people exercising hard may need the extra carbohydrate, if dose reduction alone proves inadequate in preventing hypoglycaemia. As in those on insulin treatment, people taking sulphonylureas should monitor their blood glucose levels before, during and after exercise so that effects can be recorded and analysed.

Coping with Illness and Infection

Common illnesses and infections can prove to be a particular problem for people with diabetes. Colds, flu and stomach bugs, which are usually short-lived, unpleasant inconveniences for those in normal health, can have more serious consequences for people with diabetes unless they are managed correctly. An important part of everyday living with diabetes is to accept the need to take extra care during illness and to learn, in advance of the event, what you should and should not do. Individual advice on this topic is given at the diabetes clinic and reference leaflets containing simple guidelines are also available. There are a number of generally accepted basic guidelines that should be followed, but before discussing these it is useful to look at what happens within the body during illness or infection. During a period of infection, the hormonal counter-regulatory mechanisms (glucagon, adrenaline, cortisol and growth hormone) are stimulated, with the result that fat stores are mobilized and liver production of glucose is increased, causing blood glucose levels to rise. In normal health, more insulin is produced to compensate for this but the response is impaired or absent in diabetes. Hence people with diabetes tend to become hyperglycaemic and in those with Type 2 syndrome, ketones may start to accumulate with a risk of the development of DKA. Hyperglycaemia, precipitated by illness, is likely to cause osmotic symptoms in diabetes such as polyuria, nocturia and polydipsia (excessive thirst). Fever, vomiting and diarrhoea which may accompany the illness cause additional fluid loss and hence those with diabetes are at greater risk of dehydration.

In the light of the above, the following general 'Sick Day' guidelines for people with diabetes can be readily understood.

• First and foremost, NEVER omit you insulin dose or oral medication. Unfortunately, there is a common misconception, especially if the person feels unable to eat, that the correct response is to not take the usual insulin dose or tablets in order to avoid HYPOGLYCAEMIA. In fact, as noted above, the main risk is that of hyperglycaemia and its possible consequences and omitting medication makes matters worse and may make the person severely ill. Indeed, doses may need to be increased in response to illness (*see* below).
• Monitor blood glucose frequently, ideally every two to four hours and at least four times each day. Or test urine for glucose, if this is the method used.
• Those with Type 1 diabetes should test urine for ketones at least four times each day.
• Follow specific advice given by your diabetes clinical care team. In general:

   ○ If blood glucose readings are below 13 mmol/l and there are no ketones, there is no need to adjust insulin (or tablet) dose.
   ○ If blood glucose levels are above 13 mmol/l and/or ketones are present, extra clear insulin will be needed (4 to 6 units, depending upon readings).

As the illness subsides and blood glucose levels fall, the normal insulin dose should be restored. Increased doses are needed according to blood glucose results and are not dependent upon whether you are able to eat or not. People on oral antidiabetic medication may need to increase the dose of tablets. Alternatively, clear insulin injections may be required for the duration of the illness. If in any doubt as to what to do during the course of an illness, always seek professional advice.

- Remember that even minor illnesses can cause a problem in diabetes and so do not hesitate to consult your doctor, if you are unwell.
- If you take 'over-the-counter' remedies, make sure that they are sugar-free.
- If you cannot eat normally, try alternatives such as soup, milk, ice-cream, custard, honey, fruit juice or jam as meal replacers. At the very least, sip one glass (250 ml) of a sweetened drink to replace each meal.
- Drink lots of sugar-free fluids. At least four to six pints should be drunk each day to prevent dehydration.
- If you are vomiting and cannot keep anything down, if blood glucose levels are very high or low or if there is rising ketonuria, summon medical help. You will probably need to be admitted to hospital so that your condition can be closely monitored and you can be given treatment by intravenous infusion.
- Take plenty of rest and stay at home until you feel better. Do not try to carry on as normal while ill and avoid extra activity and stress.

Flu Vaccination

People with diabetes are entitled to free vaccination against flu and this is usually carried out during October or November by family doctors. Vaccinations can temporarily upset glycaemic control and it is worth while checking blood glucose levels more rigorously in the few days after receiving the injection.

Dental Care

Regular dental check-ups and early preventive treatment are especially important for people with diabetes, since mouth infections or toothache can upset glycaemic control and disrupt eating. Many people find dental treatment stressful and those with diabetes are advised to monitor their blood glucose levels carefully following a treatment session, to guard against the possible development of HYPO-GLYCAEMIA. Your dentist should be informed that you have diabetes. Any dental treatment requiring a general anaesthetic should be carried out in hospital.

Travel and Holidays

Travelling and going on holiday, whether at home or abroad, present potential difficulties for people with diabetes. Fortunately, these can usually be prevented, or their impact reduced by careful advance planning to identify possible pitfalls. If sensible precautions are taken, there is no reason why people with diabetes cannot enjoy the same travel and holiday opportunities as anyone else. The main potential problem is disruption of glycaemic control within the normal daily routine because the person suddenly arrives in a different environment. People with Type 1 diabetes and those with insulin or sulphonylurea-treated Type 2 diabetes are probably at greatest risk. However, anyone with diabetes, especially if they already have or may be at risk of developing a COMPLICATION such as DIABETIC FOOT DISEASE, needs to take extra care when travelling or going on holiday.

It is best to obtain individual advice from the diabetes clinic or from your GP. The following is a summary of general travel advice for those with diabetes.

Travelling at Home
Travelling at home is likely to cause fewer problems, but even so there may be disruption and delays resulting in meals being missed. It is necessary to prepare for this by carrying carbohydrate-containing snacks that are substantial enough to replace meals, if required, as well as keeping diabetes treatment supplies ready to hand. It is sensible to carry some form of diabetes identification (card, necklace, bracelet etc.), especially if you are travelling on your own.

Travelling Abroad
This requires both advance preparation and extra care while away from home. There are several general preparations that you can make in advance of travelling.

- Make sure that glycaemic control is good and take advice on how to improve it, if necessary.
- Vaccinations are needed for more exotic locations, including throughout Asia and Africa. Find out what these are and have them done within the recommended time limits, bearing in mind that vaccination can temporarily upset glycaemic control. You may need anti-malarial drugs. Consult your family doctor about this and ask whether the medication could affect your diabetes control.
- Allow time for comparing quotes for vital travel and health insurance and read the small print to make sure that you get the cover that is best for you. The minimum amount considered to be necessary is £250,000 to cover all accidents and emergencies. Some countries

offer reciprocal healthcare arrangements with the UK, e.g. members of the European Union. You need to fill in and submit the form, E111, which can be obtained from main post offices and Social Security offices, which entitles the holder to free emergency medical care anywhere within the EU. You need to declare that you have diabetes on any application for travel and health insurance and ensure that the company does not operate exclusions with regard to the condition. Diabetes UK is a helpful source of advice for all matters connected with insurance.

- Find out about the nature and availability of insulin supplies in the country that you intend to visit, just in case something happens to your own. Some countries use 40 or 80 units/ml rather than the 100 units/ml used in the UK. Dose adjustment and matching syringes are needed if these are to be used. Make sure that you know what your requirements will be before you travel.

- If you are going on a long-haul flight and crossing time zones, you need to obtain specific advice about adjusting your insulin doses. Travelling east to west makes the day longer and the reverse is true for west to east. Extra small doses of clear insulin may be needed for long journeys east to west or conversely, a longer acting insulin dose may need to be omitted for travel in the opposite direction. Detailed advice depends upon the nature of your insulin regime and you should consult your clinic well in advance of travelling.

- Take twice as much diabetes equipment – insulin or tablets, syringes, lancets, test strips etc. – as you expect to need. A three-month supply can be obtained without any difficulty, which is usually sufficient for most purposes.

197

- Gastroenteritis is an all too common unwelcome addition to foreign holidays. Take antidiarrhoeal medication with you, as well as dioralyte, to replace lost electrolytes. Ask your doctor or clinic for advice. You may be advised to take a broad-spectrum prophylactic (i.e. preventive) antibiotic to guard against this. If you do become mildly ill while away, take the same precautions as you would do at home, even if it interferes with the plans that you have made.
- Make sure that you have and take with you, some form of diabetes identification and keep it on your person. A letter from your doctor or clinic giving details about your diabetes and the type of treatment that you are receiving is useful, especially if you are carrying syringes in your hand luggage. It is a very good idea to obtain a copy of it in the local language.
- Find out whether you will have access to a refrigerator where you are staying. If not, make sure that you take a 'cold bag' or other container with you in which to store your insulin and keep it cool.
- Assemble a first-aid kit to take with you containing suitable items such as plasters, antiseptic lotion and cream, foot cream, after-sun lotion, paracetamol etc.

General Advice for the Journey and for while You are Away

- Always carry insulin supplies or tablets with you in your hand luggage. Insulin will freeze in the baggage hold of an aircraft.
- If prone to travel sickness, take anti-sickness tablets before setting off.
- Inform the air stewardesses that you have diabetes. You may receive priority meal service.

- Have carbohydrate-containing snacks and glucose available, in case you need them,
- On long-haul flights, flex your feet and leg muscles frequently and stand up and walk about occasionally.
- While away, be careful about what you eat. It is safest to drink bottled water.
- Remember that heat affects diabetes control/insulin absorption etc. Test blood or urine frequently to keep a check on glycaemic control.
- Avoid sunburn and stay in the shade as much as possible; those with NEUROPATHY are at increased risk.
- Protect your feet and always wear sandals or canvas shoes on the beach. Remember that feet may swell in the heat so ensure that shoes are roomy and comfortable.
- Watch your alcohol consumption and stick to recommended guidelines. If you eat more than normal, remember that you may need to adjust your insulin.
- If you become ill, seek prompt medical help and do not delay because you are in an unfamiliar environment.

Diabetes and Driving

Most people with diabetes are able to obtain an ordinary driving licence and are free to drive. However, a number of restrictions apply, including ones that have been recently introduced by the EU. In the UK, people with Type 2 diabetes who are being managed by diet alone, do not need to inform the DVLA (Driver and Vehicle Licensing Agency) unless their condition changes and they develop complications, particularly RETINOPATHY, which may affect their ability to drive. People being treated with tablets or insulin are legally required to inform the DVLA, and if no problems are identified most will be issued with a licence which is valid for three years and is then subject to re-evaluation before renewal. This is subject to completion of a questionnaire and the family doctor may be contacted for further information or clarification. If significant changes, such as deterioration of sight due to retinopathy, NEUROPATHY causing loss of sensation, a change from tablets to insulin, or HYPOGLYCAEMIC UNAWARENESS, occur during the licensed period, then there is a duty to inform the DVLA. A doctor has the authority to order a person not to drive if he or she is considered to be unfit to do so, and in this case the DVLA are informed. In many cases, this is not a permanent ban and can be removed when the person's condition improves and he or she can then seek to renew their licence. Circumstances in which a person might be deemed unfit to drive include:

- a significant risk of HYPOGLYCAEMIA (usually applies to newly diagnosed people receiving insulin or, less commonly, sulphonylureas)
- significant deterioration in glycaemic control
- loss of sight beyond a certain point determined by visual testing
- loss of sensory perception due to the development of neuropathy
- frequent, recurrent hypoglycaemia
- development of hypoglycaemic unawareness.

People with Type 1 diabetes and those being treated with insulin are only eligible for an ordinary driving licence. They are not allowed to hold a Heavy Goods Vehicle (HGV) licence or Public Service Vehicle (PSV) licence or to drive a vehicle exceeding 3.5 tonnes.

Driving Insurance

Your insurance company needs to be informed that you have diabetes. Unfortunately, many insurance companies charge higher premiums for people with diabetes although there is little justification for doing so, since statistics do not reveal a greater accident rate for those with the condition. If you feel that your premiums are being loaded unfairly, contact Diabetes UK which runs a helpline specifically dealing with insurance.

Life Insurance and other Insurances

Unfortunately, many insurance companies extract higher premiums for life insurance from people with diabetes, but the extent of this varies and it is well worth 'shopping around'. Diabetes UK is, once again, a useful source of information as its Financial Services department has a list of companies that charge more reasonable rates.

Diabetes and Employment

People being treated by diet generally should encounter few barriers in employment, unless they develop complications or are subject to HYPOGLYCAEMIA. For those receiving insulin, a blanket ban prevents them from seeking employment in certain professions. These include the emergency services (police, fire and ambulance), train driving, airline pilot, airline cabin crew, air traffic control, working offshore, mining, working on a cruise liner, merchant navy, armed forces, post office driving, HGV or PSV driving, and, in some areas, taxi driving. If someone is already employed in one of these areas at the time of diagnosis, alternative work within the organization should be found. Diabetes UK firmly states that in most cases having diabetes should not be a barrier to employment and they not only uphold this position in a general way but will also, on occasion, take up individual cases in which there may have been discrimination.

When filling out application forms for employment, you should state that you have diabetes and the method used for treatment but there is no need to go into details. If asked about your diabetes at an interview, stress all the positive aspects such as the fact that you follow a healthy lifestyle and diet and that your condition is well controlled and does not prevent you from leading a normal life. Potential employers are generally only concerned about whether a condition will necessitate an employee having a lot of time off work and can be reassured on this point. As stated previously, it is best to explain to colleagues at work that you have diabetes and that you may need to eat snacks at certain times and may possibly require help in the event of a hypo.

Alternative Therapies which may be Helpful in Diabetes

Alternative therapies, which have become increasingly popular in recent years, cannot be used to treat or manage diabetes that requires tablets or insulin. However, where NUTRITION THERAPY is the sole approach, a naturopathic, high fibre diet including plenty of fresh vegetables and fruits, is entirely suitable. People who adhere to this type of diet are more likely to maintain a correct body weight and are at less risk in the first place of developing Type 2 diabetes. In established diabetes, many alternative remedies can help to ease specific symptoms and chronic COMPLICATIONS. These include acupressure, acupuncture, aromatherapy, Ayurvedic medicine, Bach remedies, homeo-pathy and herbal remedies. A qualified registered alternative practitioner should be consulted in most cases, rather than attempting self-treatment. Herbal remedies in particular, must be used with caution as many plant extracts contain powerful natural drugs. If in any doubt about an alterna-tive remedy, it is best to consult your diabetes care team.

Several alternative therapies are excellent for the relief of stress and depression and incorporate exercise regimes that are helpful for people with diabetes. Most help to en-courage a sense of wellbeing which in itself eases symp-toms even if it is not curative. They include the Alexander technique, autogenic training, colour therapy, dance move-ment therapy, do-in, meditation, T'ai-Chi Ch'uan and yoga, in addition to those listed above.

Scientific Research

All aspects of diabetes are the subject of intense scientific and medical research and new developments are regularly being announced. Research covers all areas of diabetes, from the purely scientific to the entirely practical, and new de-velopments reflect advances made in all these fields. They include new oral antidiabetic drugs, more advanced moni-toring, testing and insulin delivery devices, more effective screening methods for COMPLICATIONS such as RETINOPATHY and better treatment methods for complications. An example of the latter was announced in September 2002 and con-cerned a diabetic patient with gastroparesis (*see* Chapter 8, NEUROPATHY) who had been unable to eat normally due to paralysis of the gut. She had needed to be fed through a tube, had lost a great deal of weight and had several times sustained severe infections as a result of this method of feeding. A special type of pacemaker has been fitted to stimulate the damaged nerves responsible for the gut paralysis and this successful treatment has enabled the person to resume normal eating for the first time in many years.

It is hoped that genetic and other scientific research into the operation of the pancreatic cells and insulin will lead to future breakthroughs, perhaps even the prevention of diabetes in some people. Although ethically controversial at present, it is possible that in the future, stem cells derived from embryos could be grown into beta cells in the laboratory and be made available for transplantation. Alternatively, there may be a role for adult stem cells. Breakthroughs may continue to be achieved in halting or reversing loss of beta cell function.

In the meantime, the outlook for people with diabetes who have access to good medical care remains favourable and has improved beyond recognition since the early days of treatment with animal insulins. Diabetes was, at one time, the inevitable cause of premature death, but now most affected people can expect to lead a long and productive life. It used to be unheard of for a woman with diabetes to be able to have a child. Now, as we have seen, over 90 per cent of diabetic pregnancies have a successful outcome. Although diabetes remains a serious condition, both for individuals and as a global healthcare problem, it is hoped that ways of tackling it will continue to improve into the future.

GLOSSARY

acromegaly   a chronic disease that is characterized by enlargement of the bones of the head, hands and feet and the swelling of soft tissue, especially the tongue. It is caused by the pituitary gland secreting excessive amounts of growth hormone.

Addison's disease   a disease caused by the failure of the adrenal glands to secrete the adrenocortical hormones, because the adrenal cortex has been damaged. This damage commonly used to be caused by tuberculosis but now it may more often result from disturbances in the immune system. The symptoms of the disease are wasting, weakness, low blood pressure and dark pigmentation of the skin.

adrenal gland or suprarenal gland   each of the two kidneys within the body bears an adrenal gland on its upper surface. The adrenal glands are important endocrine organs, producing hormones that regulate various body functions. Each adrenal gland has two parts, an outer cortex and an inner medulla, which secrete a variety of hormones. Two of the most important ones are adrenaline and cortisone.

adrenaline or epinephrine   a very important hormone produced by the medulla of the adrenal glands, which, when released, prepares the body for 'fright, flight or fight' by increasing the depth and rate of respiration, raising the heartbeat rate and improving muscle performance. It also has an inhibitive effect on the processes of digestion and excretion. It can be used medically in a variety of ways, for instance in the treatment of bronchial asthma, where it relaxes the airways, and also to stimulate the heart when there is cardiac arrest.

amino acids the end products of the digestion of protein foods and the building blocks from which all the protein components of the body are built up. They all contain an acidic carboxyl group (-COOH) and an amino group (-NH$_2$), which are both bonded to the same central carbon atom. Some can be manufactured within the body whereas others, the essential amino acids, must be derived from protein sources in the diet.

androgen one of a group of hormones that is responsible for the development of the sex organs and also the secondary sexual characteristics in the male. Androgens are steroid hormones, and the best-known example is testosterone. They are mainly secreted by the testes in the male but are also produced by the adrenal cortex and by the ovaries of females in small amounts.

antibodies protein substances of the globulin type which are produced by the lymphoid tissue and circulate in the blood. They react with their corresponding antigens and neutralize them, rendering them harmless. Antibodies are produced against a wide variety of antigens and these reactions are responsible for immunity and allergy.

antigen any substance that causes the formation by the body of antibodies to neutralize their effect. Antigens are often protein substances, regarded as 'foreign' and 'invading' by the body, and elicit the production of antibodies against them.

atherosclerosis   a degenerative disease of the arteries associated with fatty deposits on the inner walls, leading to reduced blood flow.

autoimmunity   a failure of the immune system in which the body develops antibodies that attack components or substances belonging to itself.

autonomic nervous   system the part of the nervous system that controls body functions that are not under conscious control, e.g. the heartbeat and other smooth muscles and glands. It is divided into the sympathetic and parasympathetic nervous systems.

bile   a viscous, bitter fluid produced by the liver and stored in the gall bladder. It is an alkaline solution of bile salts, pigments, some mineral salts and cholesterol, which aids in fat digestion and absorption of nutrients. Discharge of bile into the intestine is increased after food, and of the amount secreted each day (up to one litre), most is reabsorbed with the food, passing into the blood to circulate back to the liver. If the flow of bile into the intestine is restricted, it stays in the blood, resulting in jaundice.

cell   the basic building block of all life and the smallest structural unit in the body. Human body cells vary in size and function and number several billion. Each cell consists of a cell body surrounded by a membrane. The cell body consists of a substance known as cytoplasm, containing various organelles and also a nucleus. The nucleus contains the chromosomes, composed of the genetic material, the DNA. Most human body cells contain 46 chromosomes (23 pairs), half being derived from the individual's father and half from the mother. Cells are able to make exact copies of themselves by a process known as mitosis, and a full complement of chromosomes is received by each daughter cell. However, the human sex cells (sperm and ova) differ in always containing half the number of chromosomes. At fertilization, a sperm and ovum combine and a complete set of chromosomes is received by the new embryo.

chromosomes   the rod-like structures, present in the nucleus of every body cell, that carry the genetic information or genes. Each human body cell contains 23 pairs of chromosomes, apart from the sperm and ova, half derived from the mother and half from the father. Each chromosome consists of a coiled double filament (double helix) of DNA, with genes carrying the genetic information arranged linearly along its length. The genes determine all the characteristics of each individual. Of the pairs of chromosomes, 22 are the same in males and females. The twenty-third pair are the sex chromosomes, and males have one X-chromosome and one Y-chromosome, whereas females have two X-chromosomes.

coeliac disease *or* **gluten enteropathy**   a wasting disease of childhood in which the intestines are unable to absorb fat. The intestinal lining is damaged because of a sensitivity to the protein gluten, which is found in wheat and rye flour. An excess of fat is excreted, and the child fails to grow and thrive. Successful treatment is by adhering strictly to a gluten-free diet throughout life.

Cushing's syndrome   a metabolic disorder that results from excessive amounts of corticosteroids in the body because of an inability to regulate cortisol or adrenocorticotropic hormone (ACTH). The commonest cause is a tumour of the pituitary gland (producing secretion of ACTH) or a malignancy elsewhere, e.g. in the lung or adrenal gland, requiring extensive therapy with corticosteroid drugs. Symptoms include obesity, reddening of face and neck, growth of body and facial hair, osteoporosis, high blood pressure and possible mental disturbances.

Down's syndrome   (formerly mongolism) a syndrome created by a congenital chromosome disorder that occurs as an extra chromosome 21, producing 47 in each body cell. Characteristic facial features are produced – a shorter, broader face with slanted eyes (similar to the Mongolian races, hence the old-fashioned name). It also results in a shorter stature, weak muscles and the possibility of heart defects and respiratory problems. The syndrome also confers mental retardation. Down's syndrome occurs once in approximately 600 to 700 live births, and although individuals may live beyond middle age, life expectancy is reduced and many die in infancy. The incidence increases with the age of the mother, from 0.04 per cent of children to women under 30, to 3 per cent to women at 45. It is therefore likely that pregnant women over 35 will be offered an amniocentesis test.

duodenum   the first part of the small intestine where food (chyme) from the stomach is subject to action by bile and pancreatic enzymes. The duodenum also secretes a hormone secretion that contributes to the breakdown of fats, proteins and carbohydrates. In the duodenum, the acid conditions pertaining from the stomach are neutralized and rendered alkaline for the intestinal enzymes to operate.

endocrine glands   ductless glands that produce hormones for secretion directly into the bloodstream (or lymph). Some organs, e.g. the pancreas, also release secretions via a duct. In addition to the pancreas, the major endocrine glands are the thyroid, pituitary, parathyroid, ovary and testis. Imbalances in the secretions of endocrine glands produce a variety of diseases.

enzyme   any protein molecule that acts as a catalyst in the biochemical processes of the body. They are essential to life and are highly specific, acting on certain substrates at a set temperature and pH. Examples are the digestive enzymes amylase, lipase and trypsin. Enzymes act by providing active sites (one or more for each enzyme) to which substrate molecules bind, forming a short-lived intermediate. The rate of reaction is increased, and after the product is formed, the active site is freed. Enzymes are easily rendered inactive by heat and some chemicals. They are vital for the normal functioning of the body, and their lack or inactivity can produce metabolic disorders.

Friedreich's ataxia an inherited disorder that is caused by degeneration of nerve cells in the brain and spinal cord. It appears in children, usually in adolescence, and the symptoms include unsteadiness during walking and a loss of the knee-jerk reflex action, leading progressively to tremors, speech impairment and curvature of the spine. The symptoms are increasingly disabling and may also be accompanied by heart disease.

gangrene death of tissue because of loss of blood supply or bacterial infection. There are two types of gangrene, dry and moist. Dry gangrene is caused purely by loss of blood supply and is a late-stage complication of diabetes mellitus in which atherosclerosis is present. The affected part becomes cold and turns brown and black and there is an obvious line between living and dead tissue. In time the gangrenous part drops off.

gene the fundamental unit of genetic material found at a specific location on a chromosome. It is chemically complex and responsible for the transmission of information between older and younger generations. Each gene contributes to a particular trait or characteristic. There are more than 100,000 genes in humans, and gene size varies with the characteristic, e.g. the gene that codes for the hormone insulin is 1,700 base pairs long. There are several types of gene, depending on their function, and in addition genes are said to be dominant or recessive. A dominant characteristic is one that occurs whenever the gene is present, while the effect of a recessive gene (e.g. a disease) requires that the gene be on both members of the chromosome pair, i.e. it must be homozygous.

gland an organ or group of cells that secretes a specific substance or substances, e.g. hormones. Endocrine glands secrete directly into the blood, while exocrine glands secrete on to an epithelial surface via a duct. Some glands produce fluids, for example, milk from the mammary glands, saliva from the sublingual gland. The thyroid gland is an endocrine gland that releases hormones into the bloodstream. A further system of glands, the lymphatic glands, occurs throughout the body in association with the lymphatic vessels.

globulin one of a group of globular proteins that occur widely in milk, blood, eggs and plants. There are four types in blood serum: a1, a2, b and g. The alpha and beta types are carrier proteins, like haemoglobin, and gamma globulins include the immunoglobulins involved in the immune response.

glucagon a hormone important in maintaining the level of the body's blood sugar. It works antagonistically with insulin, increasing the supply of blood sugar through the breakdown of glycogen to glucose in the liver. Glucagon is produced by the islets of Langerhans when blood-sugar level is low.

glycogen or animal starch a carbohydrate (polysaccharide) stored mainly in the liver. It acts as an energy store that is liberated upon hydrolysis.

glycosuria the presence of sugar (glucose) in the urine, which is usually because of diabetes mellitus.

Graves' disease a disorder typified by thyroid gland overactivity, an enlargement of the gland and protruding eyes. It is caused by antibody production and is probably an autoimmune response. Patients commonly exhibit excess metabolism (because thyroid hormones control the body's metabolism), nervousness, tremor, hyperactivity, rapid heart rate, an intolerance of heat, breathlessness, and so on. Treatment may follow one of three courses: drugs to control the thyroid's production of hormones; surgery to remove part of the thyroid; or radioactive iodine therapy.

growth hormone or somatotrophin or FH a hormone produced and stored by the anterior pituitary gland that controls protein synthesis in muscles and the growth of long bones in legs and arms. Low levels result in dwarfism in children. Overproduction produces gigantism in children, and acromegaly in adolescents.

HLA antigens these are the human leucocyte antigens. There are four genes responsible for their production (A, B, C, D), which are located on chromosome 6, which makes up the HLA system. One gene or set of genes is inherited from each parent and produce the HLA antigens on the surfaces of cells throughout the body. These antigens are the means by which the immune system recognizes 'self' and rejects 'non-self', and this is very important in organ transplantation. The closer the match of HLAs between donor and recipient, the greater the chances of success. If two individuals share identical HLA types, they are described as histocompatible.

hormone   a chemical substance that is naturally produced by the body and acts as a messenger. A hormone is produced by cells or glands in one part of the body and passes into the bloodstream. When it reaches another specific site, its 'target organ', it causes a reaction there, modifying the structure or function of cells, perhaps by causing the release of another hormone. Hormones are secreted by the endocrine glands, and examples are the sex hormones, e.g. testosterone, secreted by the testes, and oestradiol and progesterone, secreted by the ovaries.

hyperglycaemia   the presence of excess sugar (glucose) in the blood, as in diabetes mellitus, caused by insufficient insulin to cope with carbohydrate intake. The condition can lead to a diabetic coma.

hypertension   high blood pressure (in the arteries). Essential hypertension may be the result of an unknown cause or kidney disease or endocrine diseases. Malignant hypertension will prove fatal if not treated. It may be a condition in itself or an end stage of essential hypertension. It tends to occur in a younger age group, and there is high diastolic blood pressure and kidney failure. Arteriosclerosis is a complication of, and often associated with, hypertension. Other complications include cerebral haemorrhage, heart failure and kidney failure. Previously a rapidly fatal condition, antihypertensive drugs have revolutionized treatment and given sufferers a near-normal life.

hypoglycaemia   a lack of sugar in the blood, which occurs in starvation and also with diabetes mellitus when too much insulin has been given and insufficient carbohydrates have been eaten. The symptoms include weakness, sweating, light-headedness and tremors, and can lead to coma. The symptoms are alleviated by taking in glucose, either by mouth or by injection in the case of hypoglycaemic coma.

islets of Langerhans   clusters of cells within the pancreas, which are the endocrine part of the gland. There are three types of cells, termed alpha, beta and delta, the first two producing glucagon and insulin respectively, both vital hormones in the regulation of blood-sugar levels. The third hormone produced is somatostatin (also released by the hypothalamus), which works antagonistically against growth hormone by blocking its release by the pituitary gland. The islets were named after Paul Langerhans, a German pathologist.

ketogenesis   the normal production of ketones in the body because of metabolism of fats. Excess production leads to ketosis.

ketone   an organic compound that contains a carbonyl group ($C=O$) within the compound. Ketones can be detected in the body when fat is metabolized for energy when food intake is insufficient.

ketone body   one of several compounds (e.g. acetoacetic acid) produced by the liver as a result of metabolism of fat deposits. These compounds normally provide energy, via ketogenesis, for the body's peripheral tissues. In abnormal conditions, when carbohydrate supply is reduced, ketogenesis produces excess ketone bodies in the blood (ketosis) which may then appear in the urine (ketonuria).

ketonuria *or* **acetonuria** *or* **ketoaciduria**   the presence of ketone bodies in the urine as a result of starvation or diabetes mellitus, causing excessive ketogenesis and ketosis.

ketosis   the build-up of ketones in the body and bloodstream because of a lack of carbohydrates for metabolism or failure fully to use the available carbohydrates, resulting in fat breakdown. It is induced by starvation, diabetes mellitus, or any condition in which fats are metabolized quickly and excessively.

Klinefelter's syndrome   a genetic imbalance in males in which there are 47 rather than 46 chromosomes, the extra one being an X-chromosome, producing a genetic make-up of XXY instead of the usual XY. The physical manifestations are small testes that atrophy, resulting in a lack of sperm production, enlargement of the breasts, long thin legs and little or no facial or body hair. There may be associated mental retardation and pulmonary disease.

lipolysis   the breakdown of lipids into fatty acids via the action of the enzyme lipase.

lipoprotein   a protein that has a fatty acid molecule attached to it. They are important in certain processes, e.g. transporting cholesterol.

membrane a thin composite layer of lipoprotein surrounding an individual cell.

metabolism the sum of all the physical and chemical changes within cells and tissues that maintain life and growth. The breakdown processes that occur are known as catabolic (catabolism), and those that build materials up are called anabolic (anabolism). The term may also be applied to describe one particular set of changes, e.g. protein metabolism. Basal metabolism is the minimum amount of energy required to maintain the body's vital processes, e.g. heartbeat and respiration, and is usually assessed by means of various measurements taken while a person is at rest.

MHC (major histocompatibility complex) a group of genes located on chromosome 6, which code for the HLA antigens.

noradrenaline *or* **norepinephrine (US)** a neurotransmitter of the sympathetic nervous system secreted by nerve endings and also the adrenal glands. It is similar to adrenaline in structure and function. It increases blood pressure by constricting the vessel, slowing heartbeat and increasing breathing in both rate and depth.

pancreas a gland with both endocrine and exocrine functions. It is located between the duodenum and spleen, behind the stomach, and is about 15 cm long. There are two types of cells producing secretions. The acini produce pancreatic juice that goes to the intestine via a system of ducts. This contains an alkaline mixture of salt and enzymes – trypsin and chymotrypsin to digest proteins, amylase to break down starch and lipase to aid digestion of fats. The second cell types are in the islets of Langerhans, and these produce two hormones, insulin and glucagon, secreted directly into the blood for control of sugar levels.

pancreatitis inflammation of the pancreas, occurring in several forms but often associated with gallstones or alcoholism. Any bout of the condition that interferes with the function of the pancreas may lead to diabetes and malabsorption.

pituitary gland *or* **hypophysis** a small, but very important endocrine gland at the base of the hypothalamus. It has two lobes, the anterior adenohypophysis and the posterior neurohypophysis. The pituitary secretes hormones that control many functions and is itself controlled by hormonal secretions from the hypothalamus. The neurohypophysis stores and releases peptide hormones produced in the hypothalamus, namely oxytocin and vasopressin. The adenohypophysis secretes growth hormone, gonadotrophin, prolactin (involved in stimulating lactation), ACTH and thyroid-stimulating hormones.

plasma a light-coloured fluid component of blood in which the various cells are suspended. It contains inorganic salts with protein and some trace substances. One protein present is fibrinogen.

polyuria the passing of a larger than normal quantity of urine, which is also usually pale in colour. It may be the result merely of a large fluid intake or of a condition such as diabetes or a kidney disorder.

spleen a roughly ovoid (egg-shaped) organ, coloured a deep purple, that is situated on the left of the body, behind and below the stomach. It is surrounded by a peritoneal membrane and contains a mass of lymphoid tissue. Macrophages in the spleen destroy microorganisms by phagocytosis. The spleen produces lymphocytes, leucocytes, plasma cells and blood platelets. It also stores red blood cells (erythrocytes) for use in emergencies. Release of red blood cells is facilitated by smooth muscle under the control of the sympathetic nervous system, and when this occurs, the familiar pain called stitch may be experienced. The spleen removes worn-out red blood cells, conserving the iron for further production in the bone marrow. Although the spleen performs many functions, it can be removed without detriment and as a result there is an increase in size of the lymphatic glands.

stomach an expansion of the alimentary canal that lies between the oesophagus and the duodenum. It has thick walls of smooth muscle that contract to manipulate the food, and its exits are controlled by sphincters, the cardiac anteriorly and the pyloric at the junction with the duodenum. Mucosal cells in the lining secrete gastric juice. The food is reduced to an acidic semi-liquid that is moved on to the duodenum. The stomach varies in size but its greatest length is roughly 30 cm and the breadth 10 to 12 cm. Its capacity is approximately 1 to 1.5 litres.

syndrome a number of symptoms and signs that in combination together constitute a particular condition.

testosterone the male sex hormone secreted by the testes.

thyroid gland a bilobed endocrine gland situated at the base and front of the neck. It is enclosed by fibrous tissue and well supplied with blood, and internally consists of numerous vesicles containing a jelly-like colloidal substance. These vesicles produce thyroid hormone, which is rich in iodine, under the control of thyroid-stimulating hormone released from the pituitary gland. Two hormones are produced by the gland, thyroxine and triiodothyronine, which are essential for the regulation of metabolism and growth.

triglycerides fats consisting of three fatty acid molecules combined with glycerol, which are the form in which the body stores fat. Triglycerides are derived from the digestion of fats in food.

Turner's syndrome a genetic disorder affecting females in which there is only one X-chromosome instead of the usual two. Those affected therefore have 45 instead of 46 chromosomes, are infertile (as the ovaries are absent), menstruation is absent and breasts and body hair do not develop. Those affected are short, may have webbing of the neck and other developmental defects. The heart may be affected and there can be deafness and intellectual impairment. In a less severe form of the disorder, the second X-chromosome is present but abnormal, lacking in normal genetic material.

ulcer a break on the skin surface or on the mucous membrane lining within the body cavities that may be inflamed and fails to heal. Ulcers of the skin include bedsores and varicose ulcers (which are caused by defective circulation).

urethra the duct carrying urine from the bladder out of the body. It is about 3.5 cm long in women and 20 cm in men. The male urethra runs through the penis and also forms the ejaculatory duct.